EMERGENCY AND INTENSIVE CARE MEDICINE

SEPTIC SHOCK

SYMPTOMS, MANAGEMENT AND RISK FACTORS

EMERGENCY AND INTENSIVE CARE MEDICINE

Additional books in this series can be found on Nova's website under the Series tab.

Additional E-books in this series can be found on Nova's website under the E-book tab.

EMERGENCY AND INTENSIVE CARE MEDICINE

SEPTIC SHOCK

SYMPTOMS, MANAGEMENT AND RISK FACTORS

MELVIN C. JOHNSTON
AND
JEROME E. KNIGHT
EDITORS

New York

Copyright © 2012 by Nova Science Publishers, Inc.

All rights reserved. No part of this book may be reproduced, stored in a retrieval system or transmitted in any form or by any means: electronic, electrostatic, magnetic, tape, mechanical photocopying, recording or otherwise without the written permission of the Publisher.

For permission to use material from this book please contact us:
Telephone 631-231-7269; Fax 631-231-8175
Web Site: http://www.novapublishers.com

NOTICE TO THE READER

The Publisher has taken reasonable care in the preparation of this book, but makes no expressed or implied warranty of any kind and assumes no responsibility for any errors or omissions. No liability is assumed for incidental or consequential damages in connection with or arising out of information contained in this book. The Publisher shall not be liable for any special, consequential, or exemplary damages resulting, in whole or in part, from the readers' use of, or reliance upon, this material. Any parts of this book based on government reports are so indicated and copyright is claimed for those parts to the extent applicable to compilations of such works.

Independent verification should be sought for any data, advice or recommendations contained in this book. In addition, no responsibility is assumed by the publisher for any injury and/or damage to persons or property arising from any methods, products, instructions, ideas or otherwise contained in this publication.

This publication is designed to provide accurate and authoritative information with regard to the subject matter covered herein. It is sold with the clear understanding that the Publisher is not engaged in rendering legal or any other professional services. If legal or any other expert assistance is required, the services of a competent person should be sought. FROM A DECLARATION OF PARTICIPANTS JOINTLY ADOPTED BY A COMMITTEE OF THE AMERICAN BAR ASSOCIATION AND A COMMITTEE OF PUBLISHERS.

Additional color graphics may be available in the e-book version of this book.

Library of Congress Cataloging-in-Publication Data

LCCN: 2012942450

ISBN: 978-1-62257-485-8

Published by Nova Science Publishers, Inc. † New York

Contents

Preface		vii
Chapter 1	Pathophysiology of Cardiovascular Failure in Septic Shock *Michael Eisenhut*	1
Chapter 2	Sepsis and Septic Shock: Risk Factors, Symptoms and Management *Kenji Okumura and Alan T. Lefor*	27
Chapter 3	Septic Shock: Clinical Diagnosis and Risk Factors *Diego Saa, Fernanda Galleguillos, Catherine Céspedes and Ramón Rodrigo*	51
Chapter 4	Diagnosis and Management of Life-Threatening Infections and Septic Shock During Idiopathic Drug-Induced Agranulocytosis *Emmanuel Andrès, Jacques Zimmer, Khalid Serraj and Frédéric Maloisel*	75
Chapter 5	Sepsis: A Disease of the Microcirculation *Farid Sadaka*	93
Chapter 6	The Role of HMGB1 in Cardiac Dysfunction During Septic Shock *Satoshi Hagiwara, Hideo Iwasaka and Takayuki Noguchi*	119

Chapter 7	Pathophysiology of Sepsis and Septic Shock *Jazmina Bongain*	**127**
Index		**151**

PREFACE

Septic shock is a common and lethal condition that remains one of the leading causes of death in the hospital. Greater awareness, understanding of the condition and knowledge of effective management may decrease the mortality rate. In this book, the authors discuss the symptoms, management and risk factors of septic shock. Topics include the pathophysiology of cardiovascular failure in septic shock; life threatening infections and septic shock during idiopathic drug-induced agranulocytosis; the role of HMGB1 in cardiac dysfunction during septic shock; the epidemiological impact of sepsis and septic shock; and possible implications for the treatment of septic patients with interventions aimed at opening microcirculation.

Chapter 1 - Recently there has been significant progress in the understanding of key pathophysiological processes in the pathogenesis of septic shock providing new targets for therapeutic approaches. Key processes involved are those leading to septic cardiomyopathy and those leading to changes in contractility of vascular smooth muscles regulating global organ perfusion and microcirculation. In septic shock up to 50% of patients manifest myocardial depression as manifested as left ventricular dilation or systolic dysfunction and septic cardiomyopathy implies a worse prognosis. Inflammatory mediators in circulation in sepsis such as tumor necrosis factor, interleukin-1 and interleukin-6 cause myocardial depression. These inflammatory mediators act through G-protein coupled receptors and nitric oxide which regulate the phosphorylation state of the myocardial and vascular smooth muscle ion channels, beta receptors mediating action of endogenous and exogenous vasoconstrictors and inotropes and contractile proteins through action of protein kinases and through activation of Poly(adenosine 5'-diphosphate-ribose) polymerase (PARP). In addition to action on electrophysiology of myocardial and vascular smooth muscle myocytes sepsis may induce microvascular failure leading to myocardial cell dysfunction correlating with elevated cardiac troponin levels in septic patients, which relate to mortality. There is strong evidence that microcirculatory disorders occur in the course of septic shock with a decrease of density of perfused capillaries with sluggish or stop-flow perfusion patterns. Future research needs to explore modification of action of protein kinases to counteract inactivation of calcium channels directly and improve function of myocytes by reducing nitrosylation of key proteins with substances with effects similar to NG-methyl-L-arginine, a nonspecific NOS inhibitor.

Chapter 2 - Septic shock is a common and lethal condition that remains one of the leading causes of death in the hospital. Greater awareness, understanding of the condition and knowledge of effective management may decrease the mortality rate. Current theories about the onset and progression of sepsis and SIRS focus on dysregulation of the inflammatory response, which can lead to multiple organ dysfunction syndrome (MODS). To prevent and manage MODS, which is a leading cause of mortality in these patients, it is essential to treat septic shock. Early goal-directed therapy, which has been shown to improve outcomes, has been applied to patients with severe sepsis or septic shock. Early awareness of septic shock is important to start early goal-directed therapy. Acknowledgement of the early clinical symptoms and risk factors of septic shock are critical for the prevention of MODS. This independent review of existing literature examines recent advances in severe sepsis and septic shock, especially regarding risk factors, diagnostic symptoms and initial management for adults. Recommendations are provided for therapies that have been shown to improve outcomes, including early goal-directed therapy, early and appropriate use of antimicrobial agents and source control.

Chapter 3 - Septic shock is an important cause of mortality among critically ill patients. It arises out of a complex interaction between a susceptible host and a virulent pathogen. This interaction causes a massive release of different inflammatory mediators, reactive oxygen and nitrogen species and microbial antigens to bloodstream, and activation of different cell populations, e.g. leukocytes and endothelial cells. The result of such chaotic, uncontrolled and deregulated inflammatory cascade damages different organ tissues, which leads to multiple organ dysfunction syndrome and eventually, death. Once diagnosed the occurrence of septic shock, antibiotic and fluid therapies have been proven effective, while identification of this condition remains challenging. So, to increase survival rates and to improve clinical outcomes in critically ill patients, clinical behavior should be focused in early and accurate identification of risk factors and diagnosis. Also novel biomarkers research and development of new diagnostic laboratory tools should be promoted. Altogether, these progresses may provide a better understanding of the pathophysiological mechanisms underlying this pathology, which could result in better and earlier target-specific therapeutical strategies to prevent its progression to multiple organ dysfunction syndrome and death.

Chapter 4 - In this chapter, we report and discuss the diagnosis and management of life-threatening infections and septic shock during acute and severe neutropenia (neutrophil count of <0.5 x 10^9/L) related to drug intake. This rare event, called "idiopathic agranulocytosis", remains a potentially serious adverse event of drugs due to the presence of severe deep tissue infections (e.g., pneumonia), septicemia, and septic shock in approximately two-thirds of the patients. Recently, several prognostic factors have been identified that may be helpful when identifying "frailty" patients. Old age (>65 years), septicemia or shock, metabolic disorders such as renal failure, and a neutrophil count below 0.1×10^9/L have been consensually accepted as poor prognostic factors. In this potentially life-threatening disorder, modern management with broad-spectrum antibiotics and hematopoietic growth factors (particularly *G-CSF*), is likely to improve the prognosis. Thus, with appropriate management, the mortality rate of idiosyncratic drug-induced agranulocytosis is currently around 5%.

Chapter 5 - Regional tissue distress caused by microcirculatory dysfunction underlies the parthophysiology in sepsis. Despite correction of systemic oxygen delivery variables and macrocirculatory variables, regional hypoxia and oxygen extraction deficit persist. The microcirculation consists of the smallest blood vessels (<100 μm diameter) where oxygen release to the tissues takes place, and consists of arterioles, capillaries, and venules. The recent development of new medical imaging techniques, used in clinical investigations, has helped to identify the microcirculation as playing a key role in sepsis. Sepsis affects almost every cellular component of the microcirculation, including endothelial cells, smooth muscle cells, leukocytes, erythrocytes, and tissue cells. If not corrected directly, a poorly functioning microvasculature can lead to respiratory distress in tissue cells further fuelling microcirculatory dysfunction in a cascade of pathogenic mechanisms leading to organ failure.

Endothelial cells seem to play a central role in coordinating the microcirculatory system and promoting tissue perfusion and oxygen supply. In a pathologic situation such as sepsis, abnormal interendothelial cell coupling and an abnormal arteriolar conducted response may account for impaired tissue perfusion and abnormal oxygen extraction. Microcirculatory distress is the single independent factor predicting outcome of septic patients. In the shunting theory of sepsis, the origin of oxygen extraction deficit in sepsis is due to oxygen transport being shunted to the venous compartment past dysfunctioning and collapsed microcirculatory units. In this theory the collapse of weak microcirculatory units may result in oxygen transport being shunted past the microcirculation resulting in regional ischemia and manifesting itself as a defect in oxygen extraction. Microcirculatory dysfunction persisting for extended periods of time can act as a motor driving the pathogenic effects of sepsis.

In humans, and especially in critically ill patients, the evaluation of the microcirculation has long been difficult. Recent years have witnessed the development of new techniques that can either directly visualize or indirectly evaluate microvascular perfusion and flow. Microvideoscopic techniques, such as orthogonal polarization spectral (OPS) and sidestream dark field (SDF) imaging, directly evaluate microvascular networks covered by a thin epithelium, such as the sublingual microcirculation. Laser Doppler and tissue O2 measurements detect global decreases in tissue perfusion but not heterogeneity of microvascular perfusion. These techniques may help to evaluate the dynamic response of the microcirculation to a stress test. In patients with severe sepsis and septic shock, the microcirculation is characterized by a decrease in capillary density and in the proportion of perfused capillaries, together with a blunted response to a vascular occlusion test. Guiding resuscitation with the use of these tools may allow more complete resuscitation and improve outcomes of patients with sepsis. I will thus discuss possible implications for the treatment of septic patients with interventions aimed to recruit and open the microcirculation.

Chapter 6 - Sepsis, defined as infection complicated by acute organ dysfunction, is a major cause of morbidity and mortality in intensive care patients. Physiologically, sepsis is an acute inflammatory response against an infectious organism accompanied by a complex cascade of cellular and biochemical interactions. Recent studies have demonstrated that the inflammatory response can be accompanied by cardiac dysfunction during septic shock. In particular, myocardial dysfunction frequently occurs in severe sepsis. The extent of cardiac dysfunction varies widely, from isolated and mild diastolic dysfunction to combined severe diastolic and systolic failure of both ventricles. In some cases, it can mimic cardiogenic shock.

High-mobility group protein B1 (HMGB1) is constitutively expressed in many cell types, and localizes to the nucleus via two lysine-rich nuclear localization sequences. HMGB1 binds to chromosomal DNA to regulate nucleosome structure and stability and to control gene expression. However, HMGB1 is also secreted by various cell types during septic shock to mediate lethal sepsis. Here, we review emerging evidence that supports extracellular HMGB1 as a late mediator of experimental sepsis, and discuss cardiac dysfunction during sepsis.

Chapter 7 - Sepsis has been recognized as an important public health problem and represents a major factor in morbidity and mortality in intensive care units worldwide in any age group. Recently, the American College of Chest Physicians and the Society of Critical Care Medicine (ACCP/SCCM) reaffirmed the criteria for diagnosing sepsis in order to improve patient care, allow the enrollment in clinical trials and improve communication between ICUs. In this consensus SIRS coined the term to refer to a process inflammatory independent of cause while the term sepsis represents the systemic inflammatory response to the presence of infection.

The host response to sepsis involves many concomitant, integrated, and often antagonistic processes that result both in exaggerated inflammation and immune suppression. The pathogenesis of this condition is now becoming better understood, allowing a greater understanding of the complex network of immune, inflammatory and hematological mediators, which may permit the development of rational and novel therapies. This chapter reviews the pathophysiology of the inflammatory process involved in sepsis and septic shock, laying the groundwork for better understanding of the origin in the generation of free radicals and oxidative stress.

In: Septic Shock
Editors: M. Johnston and J. Knight

ISBN: 978-1-62257-485-8
© 2012 Nova Science Publishers, Inc.

Chapter 1

PATHOPHYSIOLOGY OF CARDIOVASCULAR FAILURE IN SEPTIC SHOCK

Michael Eisenhut
Luton & Dunstable Hospital NHS Foundation Trust,
Luton, UK

ABSTRACT

Recently there has been significant progress in the understanding of key pathophysiological processes in the pathogenesis of septic shock providing new targets for therapeutic approaches. Key processes involved are those leading to septic cardiomyopathy and those leading to changes in contractility of vascular smooth muscles regulating global organ perfusion and microcirculation. In septic shock up to 50% of patients manifest myocardial depression as manifested as left ventricular dilation or systolic dysfunction and septic cardiomyopathy implies a worse prognosis. Inflammatory mediators in circulation in sepsis such as tumor necrosis factor, interleukin-1 and interleukin-6 cause myocardial depression. These inflammatory mediators act through G-protein coupled receptors and nitric oxide which regulate the phosphorylation state of the myocardial and vascular smooth muscle ion channels, beta receptors mediating action of endogenous and exogenous vasoconstrictors and inotropes and contractile proteins through action of protein kinases and through activation of Poly(adenosine 5'-diphosphate-ribose) polymerase (PARP). In addition to action on electrophysiology of myocardial and vascular smooth muscle myocytes sepsis may induce microvascular failure leading to myocardial cell dysfunction correlating with elevated cardiac troponin levels in septic patients, which relate to mortality. There is strong evidence that microcirculatory disorders occur in the course of septic shock with a decrease of density of perfused capillaries with sluggish or stop-flow perfusion patterns. Future research needs to explore modification of action of protein kinases to counteract inactivation of calcium channels directly and improve function of myocytes by reducing nitrosylation of key proteins with substances with effects similar to NG-methyl-L-arginine, a nonspecific NOS inhibitor.

INTRODUCTION

Cardiovascular dysfunction in septic shock is pronounced and can be characterized by elements of low cardiac output, hypovolemic, cytotoxic, and distributive shock. Approximately 50% of patients admitted to an intensive care unit with hypotension due to sepsis survive, whereas the remaining 50% die of refractory hypotension or multiple organ dysfunction syndrome. In 10% to 20% of these patients with refractory hypotension, there is a clinical picture of low cardiac output due to severe myocardial dysfunction (Fernandes et al. 2008).Contrary to the adult experience where high cardiac output can be a feature of septic shock, pediatric patients with sepsis have a hemodynamic profile most often characterized by low cardiac output that results in impaired oxygen delivery and cardiovascular collapse (Pollack et al. 1984,Pollack et al 1985).This septic cardiomyopathy is characterized by biventricular impairment of intrinsic myocardial contractility, with a subsequent reduction in left ventricular (LV) ejection fraction and LV stroke work index (Hunter et al. 2010). Fatal multiple organ dysfunction in septic shock has been linked to vasomotor paralysis (Parker et al.1987). In the following review mechanisms in the pathogenesis of septic shock including myocardial failure and microvascular dysfunction are summarized and explained in their relevance for designing new therapeutic approaches. The scientific knowledge base concerning the etiology of septic shock in cellular dysfunction and cell death is analysed.

1. MOLECULAR MECHANISMS IN THE PATHOPHYSIOLOGY OF SEPTIC SHOCK

To be able to understand the changes in myocardial and vascular function in septic shock it is essential to first elucidate the basic changes in ion channels, contractile and cytoskeletal proteins and mitochondria during the pathophysiological processes of septicaemia and the role of bacterial products, inflammatory mediators like cytokines and nitric oxide.

1.1. Changes of Myocyte ion Transport by Inflammatory Mediators

Calcium Channels

Myocyte function in myocardium and vasculature is regulated by electromechanical coupling. This involves both propagation of the electrical signal along neurons innervating myocytes and the myocytes themselves and the transmission of the signal to contractile proteins. The first experimental evidence suggesting that the key inflammatory mediator of the effects of septic shock Tumour Necrosis Factor (TNF) mediates endotoxin-induced myocardial depression was provided by the observation that TNF administration resulted in hypotension, metabolic acidosis, hemoconcentration and diffuse pulmonary infiltrates. Soon after TNF administration, the amplitude of the calcium transient was decreased during systole. TNF hereby appears to depress systolic function by disrupting calcium-induced calcium release by the sarcoplasmic reticulum targeting the L-type channel-induced calcium influx. TNF's early effects on the calcium transient and systolic function were mediated by sphingosine and in addition, nitric oxide (Eisenhut M et al. 2011).

The skeletal muscle ryanodine receptor Ca2+ release channel is a key component of the excitation–contraction coupling machinery in striated muscle. It mediates calcium release from the cardiac sarcoplasmic reticulum. Nitric oxide produced by the cytokine- and endotoxin-induced inducible nitric oxide synthase during inflammatory processes in sepsis influences the contractility of cardiac muscle.

In vivo, the initial release of NO activates ryanodine receptors, but a higher concentration of NO inhibits ryanodine receptors and cardiac contraction. NO alters ryanodine receptor-binding activity by S-nitrosylation or oxidation of several classes of cysteine residues associated with ryanodine receptor protein.

Potassium Channels

Experimental evidence for the involvement of ATP-sensitive potassium channels (KATP channels) was first established by Landry and Oliver who demonstrated in an experimental model of endotoxic shock and hypoxic lactic acidosis that the injection of glibenclamide (a sulfonylurea inhibitor of KATP channels) restored arterial pressure and responsiveness to catecholamines, both of which are largely reduced during this type of shock. Several experimental studies of endotoxic shock have since confirmed these data, while subsequent studies highlighted a decrease in contractile function in response to vasoconstrictors in rat arteries incubated in the presence of endotoxin. This hypocontractility is in turn partly restored in the presence of glibenclamide (Levy et al., 2010). In the context of a systemic inflammatory response, potassium channels are important regulators of the membrane potential of arterial smooth muscle cells and thus arterial vascular tone. Activation of potassium channels results in potassium ion influx and hyperpolarization of the plasma membrane. This in turn leads to increased closure of voltage-gated calcium channels and reduced calcium influx. The resulting decrease in intracellular calcium concentrations is associated with diminished contractile function and hyporeactivity of vascular smooth muscle cells inducing cell relaxation, vasodilation, and finally hypotension and vascular hyporeactivity. The resulting vasodilation is linked to increased blood flow to hypoxic and energy-depleted tissues facilitating global lactic acidosis. KATP channels have been identified in various cell types, including cardiac muscle, neurons, skeletal muscle cells, non-vascular and vascular smooth muscle cells. Among the important activators of KATP are nitric oxide, PGI2 and adenosine which are released in septic shock. Involvement of nitric oxide was confirmed by the observation that nitric oxide synthase or guanylyl cyclase inhibitors fully reversed endotoxin-induced hyporeactivity of membrane polarisation with an effect of KATP channel blockers of similar magnitude (Eisenhut M et al., 2011).

In addition to nitric oxide ATP depletion, hypoxia, acidosis, and hyperlactatemia present during shock states can activate vascular KATP channels.

To date, two studies have studied the effects of the KATP inhibitor glibenclamide versus placebo administration in patients with septic shock. Both studies showed no significant reduction in vasoconstrictor dose requirements or any significant improvement in arterial blood pressure in patients treated with glibenclamide.

The large-conductance calcium-activated potassium (BKCa) channels are by far the most abundant of the vascular potassium channels. Their role is to induce vascular relaxation when calcium levels are elevated and thus play a regulatory role in microvascular flow. These channels are activated in part by NO and by peroxynitrite and are therefore involved in vasoplegia observed during shock states. Experimentally, their inhibition may enable an improvement of vasoconstrictor response in both animal and human sepsis. There are currently no human data (Levy et al., 2010).

Peroxynitrite can also inhibit the activity of membrane Na+/K+ ATPase. For instance, in pulmonary type II cells, peroxynitrite inhibits membrane Na+/K+ATPase activity and sodium uptake and similar effects were seen in intestinal epithelial cells.(Guzman et al. 1995,Hu et al. 1994).

1.3. Changes in Cytoskeletal Proteins

The sepsis associated inflammatory mediator TNF has been shown to disrupt cell layers by interference with the assembly of the cytoskeleton which stabilises tight junctional proteins regulating permeability or epi- and endothelial cell layers (Eisenhut et al. 2011) and is involved in regulation of ion channel function. This process is involved in hypovolemia through leakage of intravascular fluid into interstitial and alveolar spaces.

In vitro experiments showed that TNF caused marked increases in myosin II regulatory light chain (MLC) phosphorylation that could be prevented by specific MLC kinase inhibition. More importantly, such MLCK inhibition also restored barrier function in TNF-treated monolayers. TNF enhanced MLCK protein expression, and prevention of TNF-induced MLCK up-regulation blocked TNF-induced barrier dysfunction. Thus, one mechanism by which TNF causes MLC phosphorylation and tight junction regulation *in vitro* is via increased MLCK expression (Turner 2006). To develop a highly specific MLCK inhibitor, several groups have designed peptides based on the auto-inhibitory regulatory domain within MLCK. These peptides inhibit MLCK without appreciable effects on related non-MLCK protein kinases. One of these peptides was able to access the cytoplasm of cultured intestinal epithelia due to the presence of an HIV-1 TAT-like protein transduction domain. Once within the cytoplasm, the peptide inhibited MLCK. The peptide was therefore named PIK, membrane permeant inhibitor of MLC kinase. PIK effectively reduced MLC phosphorylation and restored barrier function in TNF-treated cultured intestinal epithelial monolayers.

One suggested pathway for NO action is through disruption of the cellular actin cytoskeleton through inhibition of RhoA the GTPase, which is essential for the organisation of the actin cytoskeleton and actin nitration or nitrosylation. Actin depolymerisation is known to increase KATP channel opening in isolated cardiac myocytes.

Intracellular pathways triggered by action of cytokines through G-protein coupled receptors involve the action of proteinkinase A. Protein kinase A mediated phosphorylation can influence myocyte contractility. Protein kinase A dependent phosphorylation of contractile proteins, such as troponin I and myosin binding protein C, not only enhance relaxation cycling of myofilaments but also reduce myofilament calcium sensitivity. In the phosphorylated state, troponin I inhibits calcium binding, prevents exposure of actin to myosin, and limits the force generated during contraction so that phosphorylated troponin I has a negative inotropic effect. Interestingly, it was shown that PKA dependent phosphorylation of troponin at Ser23/24 was upregulated in the myocardium of endotoxemic rats when compared with control animals. This is consistent with many studies showing that myofilament calcium responsiveness is altered in sepsis. In transgenic mice with cardiac specific replacement of troponin I by the slow skeletal isoform, PKA-sensitive phosphorylation sites are eliminated and consequently resistant to PKA-induced reduction in myofilament calcium sensitivity. An important proof of concept was achieved using these transgenic mice in a model of sepsis. These studies demonstrated that the inability to phosphorylate troponin I in the genetically altered mice substantially protected these animals from endotoxemia-induced contractile dysfunction (Lorts et al. 2009).

Disruption of cytoskeletal protein assemblies is via these mechanisms involved in weakening of myocardial and vascular myocytes and break down in epi-and endothelial barriers leading to leakage of fluid into the alveolar or interstitial space, which is associated with hypovolemia and exacerbation of septic shock.

1.3. Mitochondrial Dysfunction in Septic Shock

The electronic microscopy studies of mitochondria in sepsis demonstrated structural abnormalities in these organelles after endotoxemia or septic insult in several different tissues. Liver isolated from septic animals showed a large degree of heterogeneity, with evidence of mitochondrial swelling, loss of crystal structure and disruption of the matrix. Importantly, abnormal mitochondria were present in cells that did not show evidence of necrosis or apoptosis .In skeletal muscle of baboons submitted to *E.coli* challenge, mitochondria became enlarged and with distorted cristae and, as injury progresses, fragmentation of inner membrane was a common finding. A feline resuscitated model of endotoxemia demonstrated as early as 4 hours alterations in mitochondrial structure, with mitochondrial swelling characterized by an increase in area and rounding of the mitochondria with a substantial decrease in intramitochondrial density (Azevedo 2010). In a series of studies using near-infrared spectrophotometry, Schaefer *et al.* documented impairments in oxidative phosphorylation in endotoxemic rats. Moreover, the decrease in cytochrome redox state in one study was correlated with decreases in blood pressure and flow (Schaefer et al. 1991, Schaefer et al. 1993). Boulos *et al.* (Boulos 2003) incubated cultured endothelial cells with plasma from septic shock patients and demonstrated that sepsis causes a decrease in mitochondrial function reported as a lower rate of mitochondrial respiration and reduced cellular ATP levels. Interestingly, the authors described a correlation between mitochondrial function in the exposed cells and hemodynamic variables of the patients such as cardiac output and mixed venous oxygen saturation. Boulos et al. observed a significant depression of endothelial cell mitochondrial respiration (>60%). This decrease was prevented by pretreatment with 3-aminobenzamide, a poly(ADP-ribose) synthase inhibitor, or NG-methyl-L-arginine, a nonspecific NOS inhibitor.

These data suggest that nitric oxide and poly(ADPribose) synthase activation may play an important role in the inhibition of mitochondrial respiration during septic shock.

More supportive evidence for the role of mitochondrial dysfunction in sepsis induced cardiac failure came from a study which used cytochrome c for treatment (Piel et al.2007). Regarding the electron transfer from complex III to complex IV in the normal electron transport chain, cytochrome c could provide additional substrate for mitochondrial complex IV, an enzymatic system known to be dysfunctional in sepsis in a mechanism probably mediated by NO and/or peroxynitrite. Indeed, a recent study demonstrated an increase in complex IV activity in septic rats treated with cytochrome c 24 hours after sepsis. More importantly, treatment with this molecule improved myocardial contractility in septic animals. These results have two important consequences. First, this is another demonstration that mitochondrial dysfunction could contribute to sepsis-induced myocardial depression. Secondly, although these data require reproducibility, it may be a more concrete evidence that mitochondrial dysfunction is really connected to the pathogenesis of sepsis and not just an epiphenomenon. However, some drawbacks have to be considered in this study, since they could not demonstrate a quantitative incorporation of cytochrome c into the mitochondria and some other properties of cytochrome c may have accounted for this effect, such as its general antioxidant capacity.

1.4. The Role of Endotoxins and Bacterial Virulence Factors in Septic Shock

Left ventricular stroke work indices were found to be reduced to a similar degree in patients with various forms of Gram-negative, Gram-positive, or fungal sepsis, indicating that not factors released by each specific bacterium (virulence factors) but rather substances common to a broad range of bacteria and commonly released inflammatory mediators produced in response to bacteria and fungi determine the occurrence and severity of disease (Werdan et al. 2011).

Endotoxin

Endotoxin is released by lysis of gram-negative bacteria. To evaluate the cardiovascular effects of endotoxaemia in humans, nine healthy volunteers were injected with a bolus dose of endotoxin. Three hours after the injection of endotoxin, the typical haemodynamic pattern of severe sepsis developed, with an increase in heart rate, an increase in cardiac index, and a reduction in systemic vascular resistance. After volume loading, there was a reduction in left ventricular ejection fraction and left ventricular performance. However, it is unlikely that it is the endotoxin per se that is directly causing myocardial depression as only a minority of septic patients had detectable levels of endotoxin. The delay in onset of myocardial depression after endotoxin administration suggests that endotoxin causes the release of other mediators such as cytokines with myocardial depressant properties. It is likely that Toll-like receptor-4 plays a pivotal role in gramnegative endotoxin-induced myocyte dysfunction. These receptors provide critical links between immune stimulants produced by micro-organisms and the initiation of host defences. Activation causes the release of various cytokines and propagation of the inflammatory response. In vitro experiments suggest that the presence of Toll-like receptor-4 on macrophages and neutrophils is necessary to cause myocardial dysfunction, probably via the release of TNF (Hunter et al. 2010).

There are differences in effects of different bacteria on the type of cytokines released by cells of the immune system: Heat-killed streptococci induced greater interferon gamma but less IL-10 release than heat-killed E. coli in a whole blood model. Other investigators demonstrated that heat-killed staphylococci induce less IL-6, IL-8, IL-1and TNF from neonatal blood than E. coli. Gram-negative disease has been shown to result in greater plasma levels of TNF alpha than gram-positive infection (Gao 2008).

Monsalve contrasted the haemodynamic features of meningococcal disease (MCD) with those of other forms of gram-negative sepsis in critically ill patients (Monsalve et al. 1984).Patients with MCD had a lower cardiac output. He also found that the cardiac output did not increase in response to volume loading in MCD, whereas it did in those with other forms of gram-negative sepsis. Giraud reported similar findings of impaired cardiac performance in adults. Those with severe MCD had lower stoke volumes than did those with other forms of gram-negative shock. The lower stroke volumes were compensated for by the higher heart rates in those with MCD; the result was that the cardiac output was the same in both groups (Giraud et al. 1991).

Effects of other Bacterial Toxins

Intravascular administration of pneumolysin has been reported to result in an increase of pulmonary vascular resistance and permeability in a dose-dependent manner through platelet activating factor-mediated release of thromboxane.

S. aureus α-toxin and E. coli hemolysin A are examples of toxins which can create an inner hydrophilic cavity in cell membrane leading to endothelial cell damage and subsequent vascular hyperpermeability. For instance, S. aureus α-toxin has been shown to increase vascular permeability by producing discontinuation of vascular junctional protein. Interestingly, although both S. aureus α-toxin and E. coli hemolysin A can affect the myocardial circulation with increased coronary vascular resistance and loss in contractile function, the two exotoxins can exert different effects on myocardial perfusion. In a model of rat isolated hearts, Legrand et al. reported subendocardial perfusion impairment with hemolysin while α-toxin rather impaired the epicardial microcirculatory flow. Release of hemolysin A can then stimulate vasodilation through the stimulation of constitutive nitric oxide synthase dependant NO release (Legrand et al. 2010).

2. MICROCIRCULATION IN SEPTIC SHOCK

The microcirculation is an integrated functional system that helps ensure that tissue oxygen delivery meets cellular oxygen demand throughout the body. When this system becomes unhinged, maldistribution of blood flow and tissue hypoxia may result. Distributive shock, such as occurs during sepsis and septic shock, is associated with an abnormal distribution of microvascular blood flow and metabolic distress in the presence of normal or even supranormal levels of cardiac output. Although microcirculatory dysfunction may occur to some degree in most shock states (e.g., cardiogenic shock and ischemia–reperfusion injury), microcirculatory failure appears to be a hallmark of the septic state and central to sepsis pathophysiology. The clinical introduction of new microcirculatory imaging techniques such as orthogonal polarization spectral and sidestream dark-field imaging (OPS/SDF), have allowed direct observation of the microcirculation at the bedside. Images of the sublingual microcirculation during septic shock and resuscitation have revealed that the distributive defect of blood flow occurs at the capillary level. (Elbers et al. 2006).

The microcirculatory unit, composed of the arteriole, capillary bed, and postcapillary venule, is the landscape where most of the pivotal events of sepsis pathogenesis take place, including loss of vasomotor reactivity, endothelial cell injury, activation of coagulation, and disordered leukocyte trafficking. In rat models of cecal ligation and puncture, investigators used intravital video microscopy to demonstrate that sepsis is characterized by decreased microcirculatory flow velocity, an abundance of stopped-flow microvessels, increased heterogeneity of microcirculatory flow, and low density of perfused capillaries. As these microcirculatory flow alterations can occur in the absence of global hemodynamic derangements (e.g., absence of arterial hypotension), microcirculatory dysfunction largely reflects intrinsic events occurring in the microvessels. The ensuing microcirculatory "failure" can cause marked impairment of tissue oxygen transport resulting in tissue hypoxia (Trzeciak et al. 2008). In septic patients, microcirculatory failure appears to be a major perturbation with prognostic significance.

Severe derangements of microcirculatory flow, including the severity of initial derangements in the early resuscitation phase of therapy as well as the persistence of microcirculatory derangements over time, have been associated with lower survival. (De Backer et al. 2002, Sakr et al. 2004).

Application of microcirculatory recruitment maneuver procedures has been shown to be effective in promoting microcirculatory blood flow and correct metabolic distress in clinical studies using OPS/SDF imaging (Spronk et al. 2006, Creteur et al. 2006): Fluids in combination with nitroglycerine therapy were shown to recruit disturbed microcirculation following pressure guided resuscitation in septic shock patients, suggesting a role for vasodilator therapy in the treatment of sepsis (De Backer et al.2002, Buwalda et al. 2002). De Backer and colleagues had also shown that such disturbed microcirculation can be recruited by topical application of acetylcholine. Support of pump function by dobutamine therapy has been shown to improve micro-circulatory flow independent of improvement of global hemodynamic parameters (De Backer et al. 2006, Elbers et al. 2006).

With regards to myocardial microcirculation experimental studies suggest that generalized microvascular dysfunction is probably an important factor in the heart, as elsewhere. This could lead to relative ischaemia, microvascular shunting or flow heterogeneity secondary to mechanisms such as endothelial dysfunction, leucocyte plugging of capillaries, interstitial edema and free radical production. Growing evidence suggests that reversible mismatched perfusion metabolism areas inherent to local redistributive microcirculatory adjustment are present in experimental sepsis, suggesting an ischemic component is partially responsible for heart dysfunction. Specifically, decreased myocardial microcirculatory flow and random oxygen consumption have been experimentally demonstrated by means of positron emission tomography imaging in endotoxic shock.(Maeder et al. 2006) Abnormalities in the nitric oxide system induced by inflammatory activation can be regarded as one of the key mechanisms responsible for the distributive defects associated with severe sepsis and septic shock. Indeed, various studies have shown hemodynamic stabilization after blocking the inflammatory up-regulation of inducible nitric oxide synthase (iNOS) expression. Inhomogeneous expression of iNOS interferes with regional blood flow and promotes shunting from vulnerable weak microcirculatory units. Inhomogenous expression of endothelial adhesion molecules, such as intercellular adhesion molecules and selectines, can also be expected to contribute to distributive alterations of blood flow through its effect on white blood cell kinetics (Elbers et al. 2006).

3. MYOCARDIAL DYSFUNCTION IN SEPTIC SHOCK

Myocardial depression, defined as diminuition of the left ventricular ejection fraction, occurs in about 50% of patients with septic shock. The depression is characterized by both left and right ventricular dysfunction. Systolic dysfunction occurs early in shock with lower ejection fraction and acute ventricle dilatation. Diastolic function may also be altered, with slower ventricular filling on echocardiography and altered relaxation. Of note, inspite of the myocardial depression, following adequate fluid resuscitation, cardiac output remains high until death or recovery (De Montmollin et al. 2009).

Recent definitions recognized the importance of myocardial depression and include a low cardiac index or echocardiographic evidence of cardiac dysfunction as one of the criteria for diagnosis of severe sepsis (Hunter et al. 2010). Intrinsic myocardial dysfunction is manifest as a reduction in ejection fraction (EF), which is a clinically useful quantitative measurement of ventricular performance. Although EF is dependent on afterload and preload, assessment of the myocardium in patients with sepsis using load-independent techniques also revealed significant myocardial dysfunction.

3.1. The role of Cytokines in Myocardial Dysfunction

In recent years, investigators focused their attention on cytokines as the possible mediators of the myocardial depression of sepsis. Several types of nucleated cells produce and locally release these proteins in response to surgical, traumatic, ischemic or septic insults. Studies performed on rodent models of sepsis showed significant decreases in measures of contractility in cardiomyocytes exposed in vitro to TNF-a, IL-1b , and IL-6. Accordingly, patients with sepsis demonstrated higher levels of interleukins and complement components in their bloodstream. In a series of seminal studies, Parrillo and Kumar (Parrillo et al. 1985, Kumar et al, 2005) showed that the serum of septic patients, containing high concentrations of pro-inflammatory cytokines (notably TNF and IL-1), resulted in abnormalities in myocyte contraction and relaxation when added to isolated cardiomyocytes. It was also demonstrated that the incubation of the endotoxin with activated macrophages produced a supernatant with vascular and myocardial depressor activity. The main inflammatory mediators that contributed to myocardial depression in sepsis included ILs (IL-2, IL-4, IL-6, IL-8, and IL-10), interferon gamma, TNF and IL-1. Many studies using anti-TNF-antibodies both in humans and in animals showed a rapid improvement in cardiovascular parameters, with no drop in mortality. The administration of IL-1 in animals also reproduced the hemodynamic effects found in septic shock.

One important fact to be highlighted is that, with low doses, many times, TNF or IL-1 produced no experimental myocardial depression when administered separately, but when given together with the same doses, they produced synergism between the two cytokines, leading to the depressing effect.

Only TNF and IL-1 showed involvement of cardiac cell contraction when injected in vitro and observed by electronic microscopy, a fact that did not occur with the other cytokines (Fernandes et al. 2008).

3.2. Myocardial Cell Death

Evidence for myocardial cell death is obtained by measurement of serum levels of proteins released by myocardium after cell death. Both cardiac troponin I and T levels have been used for this purpose. Although some septic patients with elevated troponin may have either nonspecific ECG changes or regional wall motion abnormalities, on the whole, neither objective testing nor the high occurrence of elevated troponin in a population of pediatric sepsis supports the concept that flow-limiting coronary artery disease is the main cause of troponin release in sepsis. Troponin release in this population is most probably the result of low-grade cytokine-mediated cardiomyocyte injury with transient loss in membrane integrity and troponin leakage. The close association of high-sensitivity troponin T(hs-TnT) with N-terminal pro b-type natriuretic peptide (NT-proBNP) suggests myocardial origin of troponin elevation in sepsis (Markou et al. 2011).

The study of John et al. (John et al 2010) was a retrospective analysis of material from the PROWESS study: baseline cTnI data were available in 598 nonconsecutive patients from this cohort. Troponin-positive patients had a significantly higher 28-day mortality (32 vs. 14%). Elevated cTnI was also an independent predictor of mortality (OR 2.0; 95% CI 1.1–3.5). In a retrospective cohort of 121 patients with end-stage renal disease (ESRD) and sepsis, cTnI was an independent predictor of mortality at 90 days from onset of sepsis (OR 5.13) and of mortality at more protracted follow-up(180 days) (hazard ratio 5.90; 95% CI 2.06–16.9) (Kang 2009).The study by Røsjø et al. (Rosjo 2011) reported on a subgroup of patients from the prospective FINNSEPSIS study. Survivors had higher levels of hs-cTnT on inclusion. Troponin was not independently associated with in-hospital mortality but on inclusion was independently associated with development of shock during hospitalization (OR 2.45; 95% CI 1.09–5.53) and could predict development of septic shock with a sensitivity of 86% and specificity of 33%.

A correlation between troponin level and requirements for inotropic support has been mentioned by some authors, whereas others have shown opposite results. In patients with increased troponin levels, evaluation of myocardial performance during septic shock has been performed by the means of left ventricular stroke work index calculation and evaluation of systolic function by echocardiography. Consistently, estimates of left ventricular ejection fraction and fractional area contraction correlate negatively with increased levels of cardiac troponin I in both adults and children with septic shock. Serial determinations of cardiac troponin I showed a negative correlation between serum concentrations of cardiac troponin I and myocardial function (echocardiography fractional area contraction less than 50%).

However, a correlation between left ventricular dysfunction and increased levels of cardiac troponin I is not an universal finding in septic shock patients. The reason for these contrasting results has not been reconciled. However, it should be pointed out that several factors may complicate the diagnosis of sepsis induced myocardial dysfunction in humans and echocardiography derived parameters may not reflect actual myocardial contractility and dysfunction. In addition to global systolic and diastolic performance evaluation, tissue velocity imaging for myocardial strain and strain rate imaging is an important development in the field of cardiac ultrasound that provides quantitative information for analysis of myocardial motion. Increased wall strain and regional wall motion abnormalities in septic shock could be part of the septic myocardial dysfunction pattern and account for cardiac myolysis. Although regional wall motion abnormalities have been observed in some positive-troponin cases, there is no information with respect to perturbations in tissue Doppler derived myocardial strain and strain rate in septic shock patients.

Studies in unselected critically ill patients yield the consistent information that mortality among troponin-positive patients is higher than troponin-negative patients, irrespective of the cause of troponin increase. In studies restricted to patients with sepsis, elevated troponin levels have been shown to be related to the severity of the disease. Overall, these results are very similar in showing that troponin elevation indicates a worse myocardial function and unfavourable outcome (Favory 2006).

Serum TnI and CK-MB levels were measured at admission and serially at 24 h, 48 h and 96 h in children with septic shock, while baseline measurement of the same markers was taken from the controls. In total, 88% (15/18) of children with septic shock had elevated TnI levels compared with 25% (5/20) with sepsis and 6.7% (1/15) with hypovolaemic shock (p < 0.001). Serial TnI levels at admission, 24 h, 48 h and 96 h were higher in the non-survivors. There was a positive correlation between the baseline TnI levels and the predicted mortality using the paediatric index of mortality (PIM2) scores at admission (r = 0.51, p = 0.03).(Lodha et al. 2009).

Measurements by coronary sinus thermodilution catheters revealed that coronary blood flow did not differ between patients with septic shock and healthy subjects as long as the heart rate was < 100 beats/min, and that coronary blood flow was even higher in patients with septic shock compared to healthy subjects if the heart rate was < 100 beats/min. There was no difference in coronary blood flow between patients with septic shock who developed myocardial depression and those who did not, and in no patient was net myocardial lactate production demonstrated. In addition, several animal models have shown that myocardial oxygen metabolism and high-energy phosphate levels are well-preserved during experimental septic shock. Nevertheless, it is still a matter of debate whether troponin release in patients with sepsis reflects irreversible myocardial damage or reversible myocardial depression.

Whereas troponin levels are elevated for several days in patients with myocardial infarction, transient, short-lasting (*ie*, a few hours) increases in cardiac troponin levels in patients with unstable angina have been observed, which suggests that troponin leakage due to ischemia or other stimuli is possible even if myocardial necrosis does not occur. Experimental evidence supporting this theory was provided by Piper and coworkers, who demonstrated reversible membranous bleb formation in rat cardiomyocytes during limited periods of hypoxia and the consecutive release of myocardial enzymes in cell supernatant (Maeder 2006).

Despite extremely low levels of myocyte nuclear apoptosis, caspase activation has been implicated in sarcomere disarray and contractile dysfunction in various models of myocardium injury. Caspase activation participates in the regulation of cardiac contractility and its inhibition might reverse depressed contractility. TNF may induce activation of calpains and caspases that could participate in the degradation of crucial cardiac contractile proteins, including troponins. Upon activation by calcium, active calpain is released by calpastatin and cleaves cardiac troponin I at the carboxyl terminus to produce the cardiac troponin I degradation fragment. Caspases, the executioners of apoptotic cell death, also induce sarcomere disarray and are involved in the cleavage of actin, actinin and troponin T. Caspase activation participates in the regulation of cardiac contractility and its inhibition might reverse depressed contractility. Many putative caspase cleavage sites in cardiac contractile and structural proteins may be identified through data bank research with caspase cleavage motifs. The existence of such cleavage sites explains the findings that exposure of myofibrillar proteins to active caspase 3 results in actin, actinin and troponin T and myosin light chain cleavage. In experimental sepsis, studies suggested that activation of caspase 3 plays an important role in endotoxin-induced cardiomyocyte dysfunction, which is related to changes in calcium myofilament response, troponin T cleavage and sarcomere disorganization (Favory et al. 2006).

TNF may have an important role in cardiac injury through a variety of mechanisms, including second messenger pathways, arachidonate metabolism, protein kinases, oxygen free radicals, nitric oxide, transcription of a variety of cytotoxic genes, regulation of nuclear regulatory factors, ADP-ribosylation and, potentially, DNA fragmentation.

3.2.1. The Role of Poly(Adenosine 5'-diphosphate-ribose) Polymerase Activation

Activation of Poly (adenosine 5'-diphosphate-ribose) polymerase (PARP) has been demonstrated in patients who died of septic shock and the extent of PARP activation showed a significant positive correlation with the release of cardiac enzymes in sepsis as well as with the extent of myocardial contractile dysfunction. PARP is an abundant nuclear enzyme in eukaryotic cells and can be activated by certain reactive oxygen or nitrogen-derived species (hydrogen peroxide, hydroxyl radical, peroxynitrite) and DNA single strand breaks. Numerous studies have shown that the final effector of the deleterious effect of peroxynitrite on vascular responsiveness is linked to the activation of PARP (Harrois et al. 2009). PARP initiates an energy consuming metabolic cycle by transferring ADP ribose units from NAD to nuclear proteins. This process results in rapid depletion of intracellular NAD and ATP pools, slowing the rate of glycolysis and mitochondrial respiration, eventually leading to cellular dysfunction and death. Soriano et al. (Soriano et al. 2006) investigated a total of 25 patients with septicaemia on an adult ICU. During the 28 days of follow-up, 12 patients died (48%). All patients were mechanically ventilated and received catecholamines. Nonsurvivors had a more severe degree of cardiac depression than survivors. Nonsurvivors had autopsy and the myocardium was analysed for PARP activity. Immunohistochemical staining for poly (ADP-ribose) (PAR), the product of activated PARP, was demonstrated in septic hearts. There was a positive correlation between PAR staining densitometry and troponin I levels ($p < .05$).

In porcine and murine models of myocardial dysfunction, elicited by either implantation of an *Escherichia coli*-containing septic clot or injection of bacterial lipopolysaccharide, there was evidence of PARP activation in the myocardium and significant improvement of myocardial contractility in response to pharmacologic inhibitors of PARP (Goldfarb et al. 2002, Liaudet et al.2002). Further evidence was provided by human study: plasma from septic patients has been shown to induce mitochondrial dysfunction *in vitro*, an effect attenuated by pharmacologic inhibition of PARP (Boulos et al. 2003).

3.2.2. The Role of Nitric Oxide

Simultaneous generation of NO and superoxide, yielding peroxynitrite, has been demonstrated in hearts exhibiting myocardial dysfunction after endotoxemia. NO has been shown to depress myocardial energy production (Kelm et al. 1997) and peroxynitrite is recognized as an endogenous myocardial depressant factor, with a potential role in the pathogenesis of myocardial hypocontractility in shock. The direct cytotoxic effects of peroxynitrite on cardiac myocytes have been demonstrated in multiple studies. Infusion of peroxynitrite causes a reduction in myocardial contractility in isolated perfused hearts and aggravates myocardial ischemic and reperfusion injury. Echocardiographic examination of the cardiac function of wild-type and NOS2-deficient mice after infusion of endotoxin demonstrated preserved myocardial performance in the NOS2-deficient group. Further in vitro work demonstrated that sepsis-induced myocardial depression can be prevented by administration of NO synthase and guanylate cyclase inhibitors such as N-methyl-L-arginine and methylene blue. The mechanism of peroxynitrite-mediated myocyte injury involves multiple pathways, including nitration and inhibition of cardiac myofibrillar creatine kinase, actinin, and myofibrillar proteins, activation of matrix metallo-proteinases, and activation of PARP in the cardiac myocytes. For example, peroxynitrite can react with most of the components of the electron transport chain, including complexes I and III, and may mediate apoptosis by permeabilization of the outer mitochondrial membrane (Lundberg et al. 2005).

Neutralization of peroxynitrite by mercaptoethylguanidine and 5,10,15,20-tetrakis(4-sulfonatophenyl)-porphyrinato iron (III) restored myocardial contractility in various models of shock and endotoxemia (Szabo 2010). Cauwels et al. (Cauwels et al. 2009) recently demonstrated that nitrite treatment protects against morbidity and mortality in lipopolysaccharide (LPS)-induced shock in a soluble guanylate cyclase-dependent manner.

Duality of NO action in mitochondrial function has been found to be related to its effect in mitochondrial recovery. Sepsis has been reported as an inducer of mitochondrial dysfunction and, at the same time, an activator of mitochondrial biogenesis by an increase in mitochondrial genes related to recovery. Interestingly, NO has been linked to mitochondrial biogenesis since cell treatment with NO increases mitochondrial DNA, a marker of mitochondrial biogenesis, in a mechanism mediated mainly by increased expression of peroxisomal proliferator activator receptor-gamma coactivator-1alpha (PGC-1) the main regulator of mitochondrial biogenesis. A very recent study demonstrated that NOS2 regulates mitochondrial Hsp60 chaperone function, which is a regulator of mitochondrial DNA transcription and replication. Taken together, these data may suggest that the increased NO production may reduce mitochondrial function during the acute phase of sepsis for the organism to cope with an overwhelming disorder and, in this meanwhile, accelerates the functional recovery by stimulating mitochondrial biogenesis (Azevedo 2010).

4. Pathophysiology of Inotrope Refractory Cardiovascular Failure

Vascular hyporeactivity to vasopressor agents is defined by a decreased effect of a vasopressor agent when compared to the normal response due to failure of vascular smooth muscle to constrict. Vascular hyporeactivity can most often be observed either experimentally in organ chambers by exposing segments of isolated vessels to vasopressor agents, or in clinical practice by establishing dose–response curves to a pure alpha-adrenergic agonist such as phenylephrine. In this case, vascular hyporesponsiveness is defined by a smaller increase in arterial blood pressure (in patients) for a similar dose of vasopressor agent (healthy volunteers). This latter technique also incorporates other regulatory mechanisms, such as cardiac adaptation and baroreflex. Clinical evidence confirmed vascular hyporesponsiveness in septic shock, since volume-resuscitated septic shock patients remain hypotensive despite elevated levels of endogenous and exogenous catecholamines and a maximum activation of the renin-angiotensin system. Administration of large doses of catecholamines is hence necessary to increase arterial pressure. In an experimental study, Bellissant and Annane compared 20 patients with septic shock with 12 healthy subjects. Dose–response curves to phenylephrine, a pure alpha-adrenergic agonist, were established and ultimately showed a decreased response to alpha-adrenergic stimulation in the septic shock patients (Annane et al. 2005).

Hypotension associated with vascular hyporeactivity is clearly related, both significantly and independently, to mortality. The extent of this vascular hyporesponsiveness can be assessed clinically by the measure of vasopressor dosage necessary to maintain mean arterial blood pressure and by the drop in diastolic blood pressure reflecting vasoplegia (Levy et al. 2010).

Other evidence supporting reduced responsiveness to adrenergic stimulation of the cardiovascular system in sepsis is derived from investigation of the physiological oscillations in heart rate and blood pressure which are directly correlated to the response of tissues to stimulation by the autonomic nervous system. In critically ill patients, the loss of heart rate variability has been shown to possibly contribute to the progression of organ dysfunction and is associated with increased risk of death. Sepsis is often characterized by reduced cardiovascular variability and particularly by impaired sympathetic control of heart and vessel tone. The loss of sympathetic modulation of the cardiovascular system preceded shock in both experimental sepsis and clinical sepsis (De Montmollin et al. 2009, Korach et al. 2001, Godin et al. 1996, Goldstein et al. 1995).

Studies showed that intracytosolic cAMP levels are attenuated in sepsis after beta-adrenergic stimulation, leading to decreased myocardial performance. Cytokines associated with this desensitization of beta receptor signalling include IL-1, TNF, TGF beta and IL-13 (Shore 2002). In human airway smooth muscle cells IL-1 induced cyclooxygenase-2 expression and hence prostaglandin E2 (PGE2). PGE2 causes cAMP formation and it has been shown that protein kinase A (PKA) activated by cAMP can phosphorylate the beta-2 adrenoceptor and induce desensitization of the receptor by interference with its attachment with G-protein (Laporte 1998). PKA has also been shown to down-regulate beta 2 receptors by inhibition of transcription and was found to activate phosphodiesterase-4 which reduces cAMP levels (Guo et al. 2005). IL-1 mediated activation of the Gi pathway by up-regulation of inhibitory G-proteins $G_{i\alpha 1}$, $G_{i\alpha 2}$ and $G_{i\alpha 3}$ causes uncoupling of the beta adrenergic receptors from the adenylate cyclase (Mak et al. 2002). Another avenue for rapid desensitisation of the beta-2 receptor has been discovered in a rat model, where IL-1 elevated intracellular G-protein-coupled receptor kinase-2 (GRK2), an enzyme, which was detected in rat alveolar epithelial cells and is the key enzyme in rapid desensitisation of beta-2 receptors to endogenous and exogenous catecholamines (Liebler et al. 2004). Dexamethasone has been shown to prevent this IL-1 induced upregulation of GRK-2 levels. Dexamethasone also inhibits IL-1 beta induced COX-2 expression and PGE2 release making corticosteroids a potential treatment for patients with inotrope refractory septic shock.

Table 1. Pathways leading to cardiovascular failure in septic shock

Category of pathway	Mediator involved	Target	In vitro evidence	Clinical effects detected in vivo
Change in function of ion channels	Tumor necrosis factor through G-protein coupled receptors and protein kinase mediated phosphorylation and through nitric oxide	Calcium channels, ATP sensitive potassium channels, Na/K ATPase, Calcium-activated potassium (BKCa) channels	Rat arterioles, cardio myocytes	No effects of potassium channel inhibitors in patients with sepsis
Reduction of beta receptor function	Tumor necrosis factor, IL-1 beta, TGF beta and IL-13	Beta-adreno receptors		Inotrope refractory cardiovascular failure
Mitochondrial dysfunction	Peroxynitrite	Mitochondria	Cultured endothelial cells	Lactic acidosis in septic patients and electronmicroscopic findings in animal models (cat, rat) of septicaemia.
Activation of Poly(adenosine 5'-diphosphate-ribose) polymerase (PARP)	Peroxynitrite	PARP		Post mortem findings in patients with sepsis and from porcine and murine animal models
Disruption of cytoskeleton and intercellular tight junctions	Nitric oxide, interleukin-1, tumor necrosis factor	Myosin II regulatory light chain, RhoA GTPase, actin	Epithelial or endothelial cell mono-layers, cardiomyocytes	Tissue and pulmonary edema in humans and animal models associated with hypovolemia
Increased permeability of cell layers	S. aureus α-toxin and E. coli hemolysin A	Cell membrane, intercellular tight junctions		Tissue edema in humas with skin infection with S. aureus and edema in E. coli septicaemia.

CONCLUSION

Cardiovascular failure in septic shock is characterised primarily by a dysfunction of vascular and myocardial myocytes, which if the patient survives its consequence of reduced organ perfusion, is reversible. The dysfunction is caused by inflammatory mediators like peroxynitrite and to a lesser degree by bacterial toxins. It involves changes in calcium and potassium channel function, changes in beta-adrenergic receptors, cytoskeletal proteins and mitochondria (See table 1). Reduced activity of ion channels leads to reduced electromechanical coupling which together with inflammatory mediator induced dysfunction of cytoskeletal and contractile proteins weakens vascular and cardiac myocytes leading to cardiovascular failure. Breakdown of the endo-and epithelial barriers leads to loss of intravascular fluid into interstitial, alveolar and intestinal luminal spaces exacerbating shock. Compensation by increased output of endogenous adrenergic hormones may fail because of inflammatory mediator induced inactivation of their receptors on effector cells. Future research needs to concentrate on reactivation of ion channels, cytoskeletal and contractile proteins and beta receptor pathways. Such strategies need to involve agents able to change phosphorylation and nitrosylation status of proteins specifically in affected tissues.

REFERENCES

Azevedo, L.C.P. (2010).Mitochondrial dysfunction during sepsis. *Endocrine, Metabolic & Immune Disorders - Drug Targets*,10:214-223.

Boulos, M., Astiz, M.E., Barua, R.S., et al. (2003) Impaired mitochondrial function induced by serum from septic shock patients is attenuated by inhibition of nitric oxide synthase and poly(ADP-ribose) synthase. *Crit Care Med*, 31:353–358.

Buwalda, M., and Ince, C.(2002). Opening the microcirculation: can vasodilators be useful in sepsis? *Intensive Care Med*, 28:1208-1217.

Cauwels, A., Buys, E.S., Thoonen, R., Geary, L., Delanghe, J., Shiva, S.,and Brouckaert, P. (2009). Nitrite protects against morbidity and mortality associated with TNF- or LPS-induced shock in a soluble guanylate cyclasedependent manner. *J Exp Med*, 206:2915–2924.

Creteur, J., De Backer, D., Sakr, Y., Koch, M., and Vincent, J. (2006). Sublingual capnometry tracks microcirculatory changes in septic patients. *Intensive Care Med*, 32:516-523.

De Backer, D., Creteur, J., Preiser, J., Dubois, M., Sakr, Y., Koch, M., Verdant, C., and Vincent, J. (2006). The effects of dobutamine on microcirculatory alterations in patients with septic shock are independent of its systemic effects. *Crit Care Med*, 34:403-408.

De Backer, D., Creteur, J., Preiser, J.C., Dubois, M.J., and Vincent, J.L. (2002). Microvascular blood flow is altered in patients with sepsis. *Am J Respir Crit Care Med*,166:98–104.

De Montmollin, E., Aboab, J., Mansart, A., and Annane, D. (2009). Bench-to-bedisde review: Beta-adrenergic modulation in sepsis. *Critical Care*, 13: 230.

Eisenhut, M., and Wallace, H.(2011). Ion channels in inflammation. *Pflugers Arch - Eur J Physiol* , 461:401–421.

Elbers, P.W.G, Ince, C. (2006). Bench-to-bedside review: Mechanisms of critical illness –classifying microcirculatory flow abnormalities in distributive shock. *Critical Care,* 10:221.

Favory, R., and Neviere, R. (2006). Bench-to-bedside review: Significance and interpretation of elevated troponin in septic patients. *Critical Care*,10:224.

Fernandes, C.J. Jr., Akamine, N., and Knobel, E. (2008). Myocardial depression in sepsis. *Shock*, 30, Supplement 1: 14-17.

Gao, H., Evans, T.W., and Finney, S.J.(2008). Bench-to bedside review: Sepsis, severe sepsis and septic shock-does the nature of the infecting organism matter? *Critical Care*, 12:213.

Giraud, T, Dhainaut, J.F., Schremmer, B., et al. (1991). Adult overwhelming meningococcal purpura. A study of 35 cases, 1977-1989. *Arch Intern Med*,151:310—316.

Godin, P.J., Fleisher, L.A., Eidsath, A., Vandivier, R.W., Preas, H.L., Banks, S.M., Buchman, T.G., and Suffredini, A.F.(1996). Experimental human endotoxinemia increases cardiac regularity: results from a prospective randomized, crossover trial. *Crit Care Med*, 24: 1117-1124.

Goldfarb, R.D., Marton, A., Szabo, E., et al. (2002) Protective effect of a novel, potent inhibitor of poly(adenosine 5'-diphosphate-ribose) synthetase in a porcine model of severe bacterial sepsis. *Crit Care Med* , 30:974–980.

Goldstein, B., Kempski, M.H., Stair, D., Tipton, R.B., DeKing, D., DeLong, D., De Asla, R., Cox, C., Lund, N., and Woolf, P.D.(1995). Autonomic modulation of heart rate variability during endotoxin shock in rabbits. *Crit Care Med*, 23:1694-1702.

Guo, M., Pascual, R.M., Wang, S., Fontana, M.F., Valancius, C.A., Panettieri, R.A., Tilley, S.L., and Penn, R.B. (2005). Cytokines regulate beta-2-adrenergic receptor responsiveness in airway smooth muscle via multiple PKA-and EP2 receptor-dependent mechanisms. *Biochemistry*, 44:13771-13782.

Guzman, N.J., Fang, M.Z., Tang, S.S., Ingelfinger, J.R., and Garg, L.C.(1995). Autocrine inhibition of Na+/K(+)-ATPase by nitric oxide in mouse proximal tubule epithelial cells. *J Clin Invest*, 95:2083-2088.

Harrois, A., Huet, O., and Duranteau, J.(2009). Alterations of mitochondrial function in sepsis and critical illness. *Current Opinion in Anaesthesiology*, 22:143–149.

Hu, P., Ischiropoulos, H., Beckman, J.S., and Matalon, S.(1994). Peroxynitrite inhibition of oxygen consumption and sodium transport in alveolar type II cells. *Am J Physiol* ,266:L628-L634 .

Hunter, J.D., and Doddi, M. (2010). Sepsis and the heart.*Br J Anaesth*,104: 3–11.

John, J., Woodward, D.B., Wang, Y., et al. (2010).Troponin-I as a prognosticator of mortality in severe sepsis patients. *J Crit Care*, 25:270–275.

Kang, E.W., Na, H.J., Hong, S.M., et al. (2009). Prognostic value of elevated cardiac troponin I in ESRD patients with sepsis. *Nephrol Dial Transplant*,24:1568–1573.

Kelm, M., Schafer, S., Dahmann, R, et al. (1997). Nitric oxide induced contractile dysfunction is related to a reduction in myocardial energy generation. *Cardiovasc Res*, 36:185–94.

Korach, M., Sharshar, T., Jarrin, I., Fouillot, J.P., Raphael, J.C., Gajdos, P., and Annane, D. (2001). Cardiac variability in critically ill adults: influence of sepsis. *Crit Care Med*, 29: 1380-1385.

Kumar, A., Michael, P., Brabant, D., Parissenti, A.M., Ramana, C.V., Xu, X., and Parrillo, J.E. (2005). Human serum from patients with septic shock activates transcription factors STAT1, IRF1, and NF-kappaB and induces apoptosis in human cardiac myocytes. *J Biol Chem*, 280:42619-42626.

Laporte, J.D., Moore, P.E., Panettieri, R.A., Moeller, W., Heyder, J., and Shore,S.A.(1998). Prostanoids mediate IL-1beta-induced beta-adrenergic hyporesponsiveness in human airway smooth muscle cells. *Am J Physiol Lung Cell Mol Physiol*, 275:L491-501.

Legrand, M., Klijn, E., Payen, D., and Ince, C. (2010).The response of the host microcirculation to bacterial sepsis: does the pathogen matter? *J Mol Med*, 88:127–133.
Levy, B., Collin, S., Sennoun, N., Ducrocq, N., Kimmoun, A., Asfar, P., Perez, P., and Meziani, F. (2010).Vascular hyporesponsiveness to vasopressors in septic shock: from bench to bedside. *Intensive Care Med* , 36:2019–2029.
Liaudet, L., Murthy, K.G., Mabley, J.G., et al. (2002). Comparison of inflammation, organ damage, and oxidant stress induced by Salmonella enterica serovar Muenchen flagellin and serovar Enteritidis lipopolysaccharide. *Infect Immun,*70:192–198.
Liebler, J.M., Borok, Z., Li, X., Zhou, B., Sandoval, A.J., Kim, K-J., and Crandall, E.D. (2004). Alveolar epithelial type I cells express beta 2-adrenergic receptors and G-protein receptor kinase 2. *J Histochem & Cytochemistry*, 52:759-767.
Lodha, R., Arun, S., Vivekanandhan, S., Kohli, U., and Kabra, S.K. (2009). Myocardial cell injury is common in children with septic shock. *Acta Pædiatrica*, 98:478–481.
Lorts, A., Burroughs, T., and Shanley, T.P. (2009). Elucidating the role of reversible protein phosphorylation in sepsis-induced myocardial dysfunction. *Shock*, 32:49-54.
Lundberg, J.O., and Weitzberg, E. (2005). NO generation from nitrite and its role in vascular control. *Arterioscler Thromb Vasc Biol*, 25:915–922.
Maeder, M., Fehr, T., Rickli, H., and Ammann, P.(2006). Sepsis-Associated Myocardial Dysfunction* :Diagnostic and Prognostic Impact of Cardiac Troponins and Natriuretic Peptides.*Chest* ,129:1349-1366.
Mak, J.C.W., Hisada, T., Salmon, M., Barnes, P.J., and Chung, K.F.(2002). Glucocorticoids reverse IL-1 beta-induced impairment of beta-adrenoceptor-mediated relaxation and up-regulation of G-protein-coupled receptor kinases. *Brit J Pharmacol*, 135: 987-996.
Markoua, N., Gregorakos, L., and Myrianthefs, P. (2011). Increased blood troponin levels in ICU patients. *Current Opinion in Critical Care*,17:454–463.
Monsalve, F., Rucabado, L., Salvador, A., et al. (1984). Myocardial depression in septic shock caused by meningococcal infection. *Crit Care Med*,12:1021—1023.
Parker, M.M., Shelhamer, J.H., Natanson, C., Alling D.W., and Parrillo J.E.(1987). Serial cardiovascular variables in survivors and nonsurvivors

of human septic shock:heart rate as an early predictor of prognosis. *Crit Care Med*,15:923-929.

Parrillo, J.E., Burch, C., Shelhamer, J.H., Parker, M.M., Natanson, C.,and Schuette, W.A.(1985).Circulating myocardial depressant substance in humans with septic shock.septic shock patients with a reduced ejection fraction have a circulating factor that depresses in vitro myocardial cell performance. *J Clin Invest*, 76:1539-1553.

Piel, D.A., Gruber, P.J., Weinheimer, C.J., Courtois, M.R., Robertson, C.M., Coopersmith, CM., Deutschman, CS., and Levy, RJ.(2007). Mitochondrial resuscitation with exogenous cytochrome *c* in the septic heart. *Crit Care Med*, 35: 2120-2127.

Pollack, M.M., Fields, A.I., and Ruttimann, U.E. (1984).Sequential cardiopulmonary variables of infants and children in septic shock. *Crit Care Med*,12:554-559 .

Pollack, M.M., Fields, A.I., and Ruttimann, U.E. (1985). Distributions of cardiopulmonary variables in pediatric survivors and nonsurvivors of septic shock. *Crit Care Med*,13:454-459.

Røsjø, H., Varpula, M., Hagve, TA., et al., FINNSEPSIS Study Group. (2011). Circulating high sensitivity troponin T in severe sepsis and septic shock: distribution,associated factors, and relation to outcome. *Intensive Care Med* ,37:77–85.

Sakr, Y., Dubois, M.J., De Backer, D., Creteur, J., and Vincent, J.L. (2004).Persistent microcirculatory alterations are associated with organ failure and death in patients with septic shock. *Crit Care Med*, 32:1825–1831.

Schaefer, C.F., and Biber, B.(1993). Effects of endotoxemia on the redox level of brain cytochrome a,a3 in rats. *Circ Shock*, 40: 1-8.

Schaefer, C.F., Biber, B., Lerner, M.R., Jobsis-Van der Vliet, FF. and Fagraeus, L. (1991). Rapid reduction of intestinal cytochromea,a3 during lethal endotoxemia. *J. Surg. Res.*, 51: 382-391.

Schaefer, C.F., Lerner, M.R., and Biber, B.(1991). Dose-related reduction of intestinal cytochrome a,a3 induced by endotoxin in rats. *Circ Shock,* 33:17-25.

Shore, S.A.(2002). Cytokine regulation of beta-adrenergic responses in airway smooth muscle. *J Allergy Clin Immunol*, 110:255-260.

Soriano, F.G., Nogueira, A.C, Caldini, E.G., Lins, M.H., Teixeira, A.C., Cappi, S.B., Lotufo, P.A., Bernik, M.M.S., Zsengellér, Z., Chen, M., and Szabó, C. (2006). Potential role of poly(adenosine 5'-diphosphate-ribose) polymerase activation in the pathogenesis of myocardial contractile dysfunction associated with human septic shock. *Crit Care Med*, 34:1073-1079.

Spronk, P.E., Rommes, J.H., Schaar, C., and Ince, C. (2006).Thrombolysis in fulminant purpura: observations on changes in microcirculatory perfusion during successful treatment. *Thromb Haemost*, 95:576-578.

Szabo, C., and Modis, K. (2010). Pathophysiological roles of peroxynitrite in circulatory shock. *Shock*, 34 Suppl 1: 4-14.

Trzeciak, S., Cinel, I., Dellinger, R.P., Shapiro, N.I., Arnold, R.C., Parrillo, J.E., and Hollenberg, S.M., on behalf of the Microcirculatory Alterations in Resuscitation and Shock (MARS) Investigators. (2008).Resuscitating the Microcirculation in Sepsis:The Central Role of Nitric Oxide, Emerging Concepts for Novel Therapies, and Challenges for Clinical Trials. *Acad Emerg Med*, 15:399-415.

Turner, J.R. (2006).Molecular basis of epithelial barrier regulation. From basic mechanisms to clinical application.*Am J Pathol*,169:1901-1909.

Werdan, K., Oelke, A., Hettwer, S., Nuding, S., Bubel, S., Hoke, R., Ruß, M., Lautenschlaeger, C., Mueller-Werdan, U., and Ebelt, H. (2011). Septic cardiomyopathy: hemodynamic quantification, occurrence,and prognostic implications. *Clin Res Cardiol*,100: 661–668.

In: Septic Shock
Editors: M. Johnston and J. Knight

ISBN: 978-1-62257-485-8
© 2012 Nova Science Publishers, Inc.

Chapter 2

SEPSIS AND SEPTIC SHOCK: RISK FACTORS, SYMPTOMS AND MANAGEMENT

Kenji Okumura and Alan T. Lefor
Department of Surgery, Tokyo-bay Urayasu Ichikawa Medical Centor, Todaijima, Urayasu, Chiba, Japan
Department of Surgery, Jichi Medical University, Tochigi, Japan

ABSTRACT

Septic shock is a common and lethal condition that remains one of the leading causes of death in the hospital. Greater awareness, understanding of the condition and knowledge of effective management may decrease the mortality rate. Current theories about the onset and progression of sepsis and SIRS focus on dysregulation of the inflammatory response, which can lead to multiple organ dysfunction syndrome (MODS). To prevent and manage MODS, which is a leading cause of mortality in these patients, it is essential to treat septic shock. Early goal-directed therapy, which has been shown to improve outcomes, has been applied to patients with severe sepsis or septic shock. Early awareness of septic shock is important to start early goal-directed therapy. Acknowledgement of the early clinical symptoms and risk factors of septic shock are critical for the prevention of MODS. This independent review of existing literature examines recent advances in severe sepsis and septic shock, especially regarding risk factors, diagnostic symptoms and initial management for adults. Recommendations are provided for therapies that have been shown to improve outcomes, including early goal-directed therapy, early and appropriate use of antimicrobial agents and source control.

INTRODUCTION

Severe sepsis and septic shock are lethal conditions with a high mortality rate. [1-3] Before recommendations existed regarding early goal-directed therapy, there was no standard approach to severe sepsis or septic shock. [4] Until recently, there has not been a scientific basis for the identification of high-risk patients, or a standard practice for hemodynamic optimization and adjunctive pharmacologic therapies other than the early initiation of antibiotics. During the past decades, several randomized, controlled trials in patients with severe sepsis and septic shock have demonstrated significant reductions in mortality rates by using early goal-directed therapy. [5] Concurrently, antimicrobial resistance to several agents has emerged and changed considerations regarding empirical therapy. [6,7] Advances in imaging and noninvasive interventional techniques might also lead to new diagnostic and therapeutic strategies for early source control.

Some of the new approaches to manage severe sepsis and septic shock appear to be time dependent, suggesting a "golden hour" and "silver day" perspective to the management of this disorder. [8] This article is an independent clinical review of severe sepsis and septic shock. [8] The literature was reviewed and referenced through the time of the last revision and a final consensus was reached by the authors. Because of the breadth of this topic, the authors have attempted to summarize and reference the literature and comment. Specific and practical recommendations for the management of severe sepsis and septic shock based on the best available evidence and authors' opinion are provided.

RISK FACTORS

To diagnose severe sepsis or septic shock as early as possible, it is vital to recognize the historical, clinical, and laboratory findings that suggest infection, organ dysfunction, and global tissue hypoxia. Physicians should also be familiar with the risk factors for the development of septic shock (see Table1). Patients suspected to have sepsis are already in a high-risk group for the development of septic shock.

Table 1.

Risk factors for severe sepsis or septic shock
History of contact with organisms, especially meningococcemia
Medications (steroids or immunomodulators)
Disease (cancers, chronic organ disease or HIV infection)
Prosthetic devices
Advanced age
Presumed sepsis

*chronic organ disease; diabetes; liver disease; renal disease; or cardiac disease.

Both epidemiologic factors, such as the contact risk for meningococcemia, and individual patient risk factors for infection must first be considered. The presence of immunocompromising conditions due to medications (e.g. steroids and immunomodulators) or diseases (e.g. malignancy, chronic organ disease, HIV infection), prosthetic devices such as intravenous lines, heart valves and urinary catheters, or advanced age, can significantly increase infection risk. [9-13] Recently, genetic defects also have been identified that impair the recognition of pathogens by the immune system, increasing susceptibility to specific classes of microorganisms. [14] Renal disease and indwelling urinary catheters were the most important risk factors significantly associated with severe sepsis or septic shock among patients with Gram-negative bacteria. [15] Focal findings of infection should be sought with a thorough medical history and physical examination.

DEFINITIONS

Sepsis is defined as the presence or presumed presence of an infectious source accompanied by evidence of a systemic response referred to as the systemic inflammatory response syndrome (SIRS). [16,17] SIRS is defined as the presence of two or more of the following: temperature greater than 38.3°C or less than 35.5°C; pulse rate greater than 90 beats/min; respiratory rate greater than 20 breaths/min or $PaCO_2$ less than 32 torr; and a WBC count greater than 12000/mm3 or less than 4000/mm3, or greater than 10% immature band forms. [16,17] (Table2) This definition has been broadly accepted, but is somewhat limited by the lack of specificity and limited number of parameters associated with systemic inflammatory response syndrome. [18].

Table 2.

Definitions
1. SIRS (systemic inflammatory response syndrome) defined as the presence of two or more of the following
1) temperature greater than 38.3°C or less than 35.5°C
2) pulse rate greater than 90 beats/min
3) respiratory rate greater than 20 breaths/min or PaCO2 less than 32 torr
4) a WBC count greater than 12000/mm3 or less than 4000/mm3
2. Sepsis
SIRS and presumed existence of an infection
3. Severe sepsis
Sepsis and organ dysfunction*
4. Septic shock
Sepsis and refractory hypotension**

*organ dysfunction is defined as acute lung injury; coagulation abnormalities; thrombocytopenia; altered mental status; renal, liver, or cardiac failure; or hypoperfusion with lactic acidosis.

**refractory hypotension: prolonged hypotension despite a crystalloid fluid challenge of 20 to 40ml/kg.

The North American and European Intensive Care Societies proposed a revised sepsis definition. [17,19] Although this new definition is more comprehensive than SIRS, it is vague in its requirement for clinical and laboratory findings in addition to a suspicion of infection. [19] Based on this definition, sepsis describes only the presumed existence of an infection and at least a minimal systemic response and therefore would not necessarily imply the existence of hemodynamic compromise or a bacterial cause, as is often suggested by the common usage of this term.

Severe sepsis is defined as the presence of sepsis and the dysfunction of one or more organs. [17,20] Organ dysfunction can be defined as acute lung injury; coagulation abnormalities; thrombocytopenia; altered mental status; renal, liver, or cardiac failure; or hypoperfusion with lactic acidosis. [19-21] Septic shock is defined as the presence of sepsis and refractory hypotension despite a crystalloid fluid challenge of 20 to 40 mL/kg. [17,19,20] Bacteremia is the presence of viable bacteria in the blood and is found only in about 50% of cases of severe sepsis and septic shock, whereas 20% to 30% of patients will have no microbial cause identified from any source. [1,16] According to the current understanding of the pathophysiology of sepsis and the types of patients enrolled in pivotal clinical trials, severe sepsis and septic shock are closely related. Septic shock can also be viewed as severe sepsis accompanied by cardiovascular failure.

PATHOGENESIS

Serial pathological events are responsible for a transition from sepsis to septic shock. The initial reaction to infection is a neurohumoral, generalized anti-inflammatory response, which begins with the activation of monocytes, macrophages, and neutrophils that interact with endothelial cells through numerous pathogen recognition receptors. [22] A further host response includes the mobilization of plasma substances as a result of this cellular activation and endothelial disruption. The vascular endothelium seems to be the predominant site of these reactions, which causes microvascular injury, thrombosis, and a loss of endothelial integrity, resulting in tissue ischemia. [23] These disruptions are responsible for the dysfunction of various organs and global tissue hypoxia that accompany severe sepsis or septic shock.

Decreased oxygen delivery and increased consumption at the cell and tissue level, being the principal components of oxygen transport physiology, become requisite to an understanding of the pathogenic, diagnostic, and therapeutic implications of global tissue hypoxia. Oxygen is delivered to the tissue, and a certain fraction extracted at the tissue level, with the remainder returning to the venous circulation. The product of systemic oxygen delivery and the percentage of oxygen extracted by the tissues, normally 25%, is the systemic oxygen consumption. The balance between systemic oxygen delivery and consumption is reflected by the mixed venous hemoglobin oxygen saturation (SvO2).

One of the most important events leading to morbidity and mortality in patients with severe sepsis or septic shock is the development of cardiovascular insufficiency and resulting global tissue hypoxia. [1,24-26] Global tissue hypoxia develops from multiple mechanisms causing cardiovascular insufficiency, resulting in further endothelial cell activation and generalized inflammation. [27-31] Even in the presence of a normal or high cardiac output in severe sepsis or septic shock, hypoperfusion abnormalities can still exist, which is called "distributive shock". This is a state of either systemic or regional hypoperfusion as a result of derangements in blood flow distribution and loss of vasoregulatory control to the vascular beds. In addition, as a result of effects of inflammatory mediators, myocardial depression reflecting a hypodynamic state with low cardiac output can be the predominant hemodynamic feature in up to 15% of patients presenting with severe sepsis or septic shock and may be especially profound in patients with preexisting cardiac disease. [32,33]

To recognize global tissue hypoxia, it is helpful to measure the central venous oxygen saturation (ScvO2), which is usually 5% to 7% higher than SvO2 with very good correlation coefficients, and serum lactate level. [34-45] Global tissue hypoxia can occur despite the presence of stable vital signs. [46] Sepsis causes impairment of oxygen delivery, and the bioenergetics of cellular oxygen extraction and use or respiration may also be impaired. [47,48] This cytopathic hypoxia can manifest with a normal or high SvO2 as well as lactic acidosis. This hypoxia and lactic acidosis cause hyperventilation to activate the central respiratory receptors, which may be related to the state of sepsis, resulting in respiratory alkalosis in the early stages of sepsis.

SYMPTOMS

The hallmark clinical finding for infection is fever, but general thresholds for abnormally high or low temperatures are based on studies of various populations and can vary among individuals and time of day. [49] The elderly and patients with myocardial dysfunction or shock tend to have lower temperatures than younger adults [50, 51]. Oral temperature above 37.2°C (99.0°F) (or rectal temperature above 37.5°C (99.5°F)) should be considered a fever in the elderly. [49] Temperature less than 36°C (96.8°F) is associated with the presence of severe infection [17, 52]. Some patients may present without fever, and develop fever during their evaluation or after resuscitation. Other systemic inflammatory response syndrome criteria, such as tachycardia and tachypnea, were entry criteria in pivotal trials and when accompanied by a source of infection, ill appearance, or hypotension should trigger an expedited emergent evaluation for the presence of severe sepsis or septic shock.

Certain laboratory value abnormalities are among the criteria for sepsis and therefore, various tests are recommended when a severe infection is suspected. These include a CBC with differential, standard chemistry panel including bicarbonate, creatinine, liver enzymes, lactate, and coagulation studies. Leukocytosis, neutrophilia, and premature granulocytes are typically associated with the presence of bacterial infection but have poor sensitivity and specificity and, thus, cannot be used alone to either exclude or confirm the diagnosis of bacterial infection.[53-58] The presence of Döhle's bodies, toxic granules, and vacuoles heightens the likelihood of bacterial infection.[53] Overwhelming severe sepsis or septic shock can also be associated with leukopenia and neutropenia. Initial measurement of hemoglobin and hematocrit levels would commonly reveal hemoconcentration because of significant hypovolemia, and fluid resuscitation is expected to decrease RBC concentrations. Since a hematocrit level less than 30% is a specific criterion for transfusion in many resuscitation protocols, repeated evaluations are recommended. Thrombocytopenia, regardeded as one of the signs of disseminated intravascular coagulation, is an independent predictor of multiple organ failure and poor outcome. [59-61] A standard chemistry panel that reveals metabolic acidosis may represent the presence of lactic acidosis. Elevation of serum lactate will not always be accompanied by a low bicarbonate level or increased anion gap, and the lactate level should also be measured if severe sepsis is suspected. [62, 63] Increased lactate levels in initial evaluations accompanied with infection and upward trends in lactate levels are associated with poor prognosis and may be used to guide response to therapy. [64-67]

More than 80 biological markers of sepsis (e.g. C-reactive protein, interleukin 6, procalcitonin and protein C etc.) have been investigated both for their diagnostic and prognostic capabilities. [68,69] Interleukin-6 may be one of the inflammatory makers related to the prognosis of the patients. [68] In general, abnormal levels of these markers have been associated with increased morbidity and mortality. However, lack of availability, long result turnaround times, and nonstandardized assays and cutoff values limit their practical use. The plasma concentration of soluble TREM-1 (triggering receptor expressed on myeloid cells), a member of the immunoglobulin superfamily that is specifically up-regulated in the presence of bacterial products, is increased in patients with sepsis and may provide prognostic information in patients with sepsis. [70-72] Evaluation of the clinical usefulness of both procalcitonin and TREM-1 is still in its earliest stages and should be considered preliminary. Until additional clinical investigations have been performed, we do not suggest the routine use of either.

Although establishing a definitive microbial cause of severe sepsis or septic shock may be difficult during the initial evaluation, identification of the organism(s) and antimicrobial susceptibilities are critical to the subsequent management. Appropriate cultures before antimicrobial treatment to look for the cause optimize pathogen identification. Blood cultures will be positive in about 50% of patients with severe sepsis or septic shock. [24] Patients suspected to have severe sepsis or septic shock should have at least two (2 full volume sets) blood cultures obtained. For a suspected indwelling line infection, the catheter should be removed as soon as possible and the tip cultured. Selection of other culture sites should be based on the clinical scenario. The most common sites of infection causing severe sepsis or septic shock are pulmonary, genitourinary, intraabdominal, skin, and indwelling lines. At the present time, non-culture based microbiologic testing (e.g., antigen testing, polymerase chain reaction) is not useful in the routine evaluation of patients. [73, 74]

MANAGEMENT

Results of the Surviving Sepsis Campaign (SSC), originally launched in 2002, have been widely accepted. The primary method used to achieve this goal was the development of evidence-based sepsis care guidelines published in 2004 and revised in 2008. [20] In order to achieve stabilization after the diagnosis of sepsis, the management of patients with sepsis is influenced more by appropriate treatment with antibiotics and fluids than by specific intensive care measures. Therefore, the early administration of antibiotics and fluid intervention should never be delayed. The early aggressive treatment of septic shock is well documented in the SSC. The keys to effective treatment are infection control, hemodynamic stabilization, and modulation of the septic response.

EARLY MANAGEMENT

The first priority in any patient with severe sepsis or septic shock is stabilization of the airway and assurance of adequate breathing. Next, perfusion to the peripheral tissues should be restored [20,75]. These principles are similar to the "ABCs" of basic trauma care. To stabilize respiration, supplemental oxygen should be given to patients with sepsis and oxygenation monitored continuously with pulse oximetry. Intubation and mechanical ventilation may be necessary to support the increased work of breathing that typically accompanies sepsis, or for airway protection since encephalopathy and altered mental status frequently complicate sepsis [76,77]. Chest radiographs and arterial blood gas analysis should be obtained following initial stabilization to diagnose frequent pulmonary complications such as acute lung injury (ALI) or acute respiratory distress syndrome (ARDS).

Once the patient's respiratory status has been stabilized, the adequacy of perfusion should be assessed. Hypotension a common indicator that perfusion is inadequate, and the blood pressure should be assessed early and often, and an arterial catheter may be required. Critical hypoperfusion can also occur in the absence of hypotension, especially during the early stages of sepsis. Clinical evidence of impaired perfusion should be identified and sought in all patients with sepsis. Common signs of hypoperfusion include cool, vasoconstricted skin due to redirection of blood flow to core organs (although warm, flushed skin may be present in the early phases of sepsis), obtundation or restlessness, oliguria or anuria, and lactic acidosis. [20,47-49] These findings may be modified by preexisting disease or medications because elderly patients, diabetic patients, and patients who take beta-blockers may not exhibit an appropriate tachycardia as blood pressure falls. Patients with chronic hypertension may develop critical hypoperfusion at a higher blood pressure than healthy patients (ie, relative hypotension).

After the initial assessment, a central venous catheter (CVC) should be placed in most patients with severe sepsis or septic shock. A CVC can be used to infuse intravenous fluids, infuse medications, infuse blood products, and draw blood. In addition, it can be used for hemodynamic monitoring by measuring the central venous pressure (CVP) and the central venous oxyhemoglobin saturation (ScvO2). In one clinical trial, treatment of septic shock guided by the ScvO2 reduced mortality. [5] Pulmonary artery catheters should not be used in the routine management of patients with severe sepsis or septic shock because they has shown to be a poor predictor of fluid responsiveness in sepsis and the SvO2 is similar to the ScvO2, which can be obtained from a CVC. [78, 79] In addition, pulmonary artery catheters are associated with complications and have not been shown to improve outcome. [78, 79, 80, 81] In select patients, a pulmonary artery catheter may be useful.

Once it has been determined tthat hypoperfusion is present, early restoration of perfusion is necessary to prevent or limit multiple organ dysfunction, as well as to reduce mortality. Hypoperfusion results from the loss of plasma volume into the interstitial space, decreased vascular tone, and myocardial depression. The increase in the cardiac output that is necessary to compensate for the diminished vascular tone may be limited by myocardial depression. Resuscitation of the circulation should target a central or mixed venous oxyhemoglobin saturation (ScvO2 or SvO2, respectively) of ≥70 percent. [5, 20] Other common goals include a central venous pressure (CVP)

8 to 12 mmHg, a mean arterial pressure (MAP) ≥65 mmHg, and a urine output ≥0.5 mL/kg per hour, although these targets have not been well studied.

Lactate clearance has been evaluated as a potential substitute for ScvO2 as the target of resuscitation. [82] There was no difference in hospital mortality, length of stay, ventilator-free days, or incidence of multiorgan failure, suggesting that lactate clearance criteria may be an acceptable alternative to ScvO2 criteria. In early sepsis, most lactate is probably a byproduct of anaerobic metabolism due to organ hypoperfusion. Supporting this view, early goal-directed therapy decreases lactate levels faster than conventional therapy. [5] After the restoration of perfusion, however, elevated lactate levels are probably due to causes other than anaerobic metabolism and further increasing oxygen delivery to the peripheral tissues is unlikely to decrease its levels. [83] As a result, serum lactate levels are generally unhelpful following restoration of perfusion, but a rising lactate level should prompt reevaluation of perfusion.

We consider the numeric goals for CVP, MAP, and urine output to be guidelines and always consider additional clinical signs of hypoperfusion when assessing the patient's response to a therapy and need for more of a therapy. These include blood pressure, arterial lactate, urine output, creatinine, platelet count, Glasgow coma scale score, serum bilirubin, liver enzymes, oxygenation (ie, arterial oxygen tension or oxyhemoglobin saturation), and gut function. Gastric tonometry may also be helpful, if available. Gastric tonometry indirectly measures perfusion to the gut by estimating the gastric mucosal PCO2. It can be used to detect gut hypoxia by calculating the gastric to arterial PCO2 gap. [84, 85] But, gastric tonometry is not widely available and it is uncertain whether it can successfully guide therapy. Reevaluation is indicated if any of these parameters worsen or fail to improve. Additional studies and clinical experience are needed.

Ongoing Management

Infection control is vital to maximize the chances of long-term survival. Appropriate antibiotics must be given within the first hour of recognition of sepsis after obtaining various cultures. A delay in appropriate antibiotic treatment leads to a poorer outcome. For every hour lost, mortality climbs by 9%. [20] A focus of infection must be assessed immediately. The patient should be evaluated, when source control is required, and effective intervention should be performed with the least physiologic insult. Prompt identification and treatment of the primary site or sites of infection are essential. [1, 24, 86] A careful history and physical examination may yield clues to the source of sepsis and help guide microbiologic evaluation. Gram stain of material from sites of possible infection may give early clues to the etiology of infection while cultures are incubating. Potentially infected vascular access devices should be removed (if possible), abscesses should be drained, and extensive soft tissue infections should be debrided or amputated.

Glycemic control is an important aspect of sepsis management. In the past, insulin drips were considered for diabetic patients only and the fear of hypoglycemia led to accept glucose levels of 200mg/dl. In SSC 2004, maintaining appropriate glucose levels with continuous insulin infusion was recommended. However, tight glycemic control has a risk of hypoglycemia, as revealed by two randomized control studies. [87, 88] Hypoglycemia increases mortality and should be avoided. The NICE-SUGAR trial showed a higher mortality rate with tight glycemic control. [89] Hyperglycemia also increased the risk of infection, but careful attention must be paid to prevent and detect severe hypoglycemia to prevent adverse outcomes.

No evidence exists to support the use of human recombinant activated protein C (APC) for treating patients with severe sepsis or septic shock. Additionally, APC is associated with a higher risk of bleeding. Unless additional RCTs provide evidence of a treatment effect, policy-makers, clinicians and academics should not promote the use of APC. [90] Effective treatment of the active infection is essential to success the treatment of severe sepsis and septic shock.

Source control (physical measures undertaken to eradicate a focus of infection and eliminate or treat ongoing microbial proliferation and infection) should be undertaken since undrained foci of infection may not respond to antibiotics alone. Intravenous antibiotic therapy should be initiated immediately after obtaining appropriate cultures, since early initiation of antibiotic therapy is associated with lower mortality. [91] The choice of antibiotics can be complex and should consider the patient's history, comorbidities, clinical context, Gram stain data, and local resistance patterns. [13, 92, 93, 94] Poor outcomes are associated with inadequate or inappropriate antimicrobial therapy (ie, treatment with antibiotics to which the pathogen is later shown to be resistant in vitro) [94-100]. They are also associated with delays in initiating antimicrobial therapy, even short delays (e.g., one hour).

When the potential pathogen or infection source is not immediately obvious, we favor broad-spectrum antibiotic coverage directed against both gram-positive and gram-negative bacteria. A detailed history, careful physical examination and appropriate imaging studies are essential to identify the source of infection. Considering local susceptibility patterns, an empiric antibiotic regimen should be used. Staphylococcus aureus is associated with significant morbidity if not treated early in the course of infection. [101]. The duration of therapy is typically 7 to 10 days, although longer courses may be appropriate in patients who have a slow clinical response, an undrainable focus of infection, or immunologic deficiencies [20].

Glucocorticoids have long been investigated as therapeutic agents in sepsis because the pathogenesis of sepsis involves an intense and potentially deleterious host inflammatory response. Steroid use in sepsis had a renaissance when a multicenter randomized clinical trial in 2002 showed a survival advantage with no difference in adverse events. [102] SSC 2004 recommended the use of low dose intravenous corticosteroids for septic patients who require vasopressors after fluid resuscitation. After the publication of the 2004 guidelines, significantly different results were found in CORTICUS. [103] In light of these two conflicting studies, the SSC recommendations give relatively tempered guidelines. Intravenous hydrocortisone should be considered only in septic shock patients who are only poorly responsive to fluid resuscitation and vasopressor therapies. Because there was no difference in response to steroids between responders and non-responders to an ACTH stimulation test, this test should not be used to select patients to receive steroids. [20] This represents a much less enthusiastic endorsement for the use of this therapy.

There is consensus that nutrition support improves outcomes in critically ill patients, such as body weight and mid-arm muscle mass. However, it is uncertain whether nutrition support improves important clinical outcomes (eg, duration of mechanical ventilation, length of stay, mortality), or when nutrition support should be initiated. [104,105,106] In addition, although there are many tools to assess the patients' nutrition status, there is no widely accepted tool to determine the nutrition status. [107, 108] Nutritional risk screening (NRS) may be useful. [107] According to guidelines, the patients' nutritional status should be categorized. (Table 3) A high-risk of malnutrition should be regarded as the presence of one or more of the following: a body mass index (BMI) less than 18.5 kg/m2; history of unintentional weight loss (5 % of body weight over 1 month, or 10 % of body weight over 6 months); prolonged period of poor nutrition intake; or chronic organ disease (such as COPD, diabetes, liver disease, renal disease, cardiac disease, or etc.)[107] Nutritional surrogates (eg, albumin, prealbumin/transthyretin) might be useful along with other indicators, but should not be used to diagnose malnutrition in critically ill patients. [109]

Table 3.

Assessment of Nutrition Status: Malnutrition
A history of unintentional weigh loss (5 % of BW* over 1 month, or 10 % of BW over 6 months)
Prolonged period of poor nutritional intake
Chronic organ disease**
a body mass index (BMI) less than 18.5 kg/m2

A high-risk for malnutrition should be regarded as the presence of one or more of the above. *BW; body weight.
**chronic organ disease; diabetes; liver disease; renal disease; or cardiac disease.

Table 4.

Overall recommendations for the management of septic shock
1 Early recognition and early goal-directed therapy
2 Seeking a source of infection with aggressive source control
3 Appropriate cultures and early empiric antibiotic therapy
4 Glucocorticoids should not be used routinely
5 Appropriate glycemic control, avoiding excessive hyper- or hypo-glycemia
6 Activated protein C should not be used
7 Nutrition support using an appropriate route based on the patient's nutrition status.
8 Effective protocols to treat severe sepsis or septic shock to assure appropriate comprehensive management

Critically ill patients without contraindications to enteral nutrition should receive early enteral nutrition. [104,110,111] For adequately nourished patients who have contraindications to enteral nutrition, the use of parenteral nutrition cannot be recommended. However, malnourished patients who have contraindications to receiving enteral nutrition, should be considered for parenteral nutrition. [112-114] Appropriate required calories are still debated, but overfeeding should be avoided. [114,115].

Based on previous studies, sepsis treatment protocols may improve overall outcomes [116-118] It has been shown that implementation of a standardized hospital order set as part of sepsis protocols was associated with greater likelihood that the initial antibiotic regimen targeted the culprit microorganism, shorter hospital stay, and lower 28-day mortality, compared to historical controls. [118] In septic shock, the activation of the sepsis response team may increase compliance with the process of care and reduce the hospital mortality rate. [119]

RECOMMENDATIONS

Based on existing literature, these are the following recommendations are provided regarding therapies that have been shown to improve outcomes:

1. Early recognition is the key to treatment of severe sepsis or septic shock. Therefore, when patients are suspected to have these conditions, early goal-directed therapy should be instituted as soon as possible.
2. A source of infection should be sought through clinical evaluation, urinalysis, chest radiography, and other appropriate imaging studies. According to the site of infection, source control should be pursued aggressively.
3. Appropriate cultures (including blood, urine, and site specific) should be obtained and early empiric antibiotics started as soon as possible.
4. Glucocorticoids should not be used routinely and should be considered only in patents with refractory septic shock.
5. Glycemic control is important for sepsis management. Hyperglycemia increases the risk of infection, but careful attention must be paid to prevent and detect severe hypoglycemia to reduce morbidity and mortality.
6. Activated protein C should not be used because there is no evidence to support this therapy for patients with severe sepsis or septic shock.
7. Nutrition support should be given using an appropriate route based on the patients' nutrition status.
8. To successfully accomplish comprehensive management, effective protocols should be used to treat patients with severe sepsis or septic shock.

REFERENCES

[1] Rangel-Frausto MS, Pittet D, Costigan M, et al. The natural history of the systemic inflammatory response syndrome (SIRS): a prospective study. *JAMA*. 1995;273:117-123.

[2] Angus DC, Wax RS. Epidemiology of sepsis: an update. *Crit. Care Med.* 2001;29:S109-S116.

[3] Angus DC, Linde-Zwirble WT, Lidicker J, et al. Epidemiology of severe sepsis in the United States: analysis of incidence, outcome, and associated costs of care. *Crit. Care Med.* 2001;29:1303-1310.

[4] Houck PM, Bratzler DW, Nsa W, et al. Timing of antibiotic administration and outcomes for Medicare patients hospitalized with community-acquired pneumonia. *Arch. Intern. Med.* 2004;164:637-644.

[5] Rivers E, Nguyen B, Havstad S, et al. Early goal-directed therapy in the treatment of severe sepsis and septic shock. *N. Engl. J. Med.* 2001;345:1368-1377.

[6] Whitney CG, Farley MM, Hadler J, et al. Increasing prevalence of multidrug-resistant Streptococcus pneumoniae in the United States. *N. Engl. J. Med.* 2000;343:1917-1924.

[7] Burke JP. Infection control: a problem for patient safety. *N. Engl. J. Med.* 2003;348:651-656.

[8] Blow O, Magliore L, Claridge JA, et al. The golden hour and the silver day: detection and correction of occult hypoperfusion within 24 hours improves outcome from major trauma. *J. Trauma.* 1999;47:964-969.

[9] Martin GS, Mannino DM, Eaton S, et al.. The epidemiology of sepsis in the United States from 1979 through 2000. *N. Engl. J. Med* 2003; 348:1546–1554.

[10] Annane D, Aegerter P, Jars-Guincestre MC, et al. Current epidemiology of septic shock: the CUB-Rea Network. *Am. J. Respir. Crit. Care Med.* 2003; 1687: 165–172.

[11] Alberti C, Brun-Buisson C, Burchardi H, et al. Epidemiology of sepsis and infection in ICU patients from an international multicentre cohort study. *Intensive Care Med.* 2002; 28: 108–121.

[12] Martin GS, Mannino DM, Moss M. The effect of age on the development and outcome of adult sepsis. *Crit. Care Med.* 2006;34:15-21.

[13] Okumura K, Shoji F, Yoshida M, et al. *Journal of Medical Case Reports* 2011; 5:499-501.

[14] Netea MG, van der Meer JW. Immunodeficiency and genetic defects of pattern-recognition receptors. *N. Engl. J. Med.* 2011;364:60-70.

[15] Kanq Cl, Song JH, Chung DR, et al.Risk factors and pathogenic significance of severe sepsis and septic shock in 2286 patients with gram-negative bacteremia. *J. Infect.* 2011;62:26-33.

[16] American College of Chest Physicians/Society of Critical Care Medicine Consensus Conference. Definitions for sepsis and organ failure and

guidelines for the use of innovative therapies in sepsis. *Crit. Care Med.* 1992;20:864-874.
[17] Annane, D, Bellissant, E, Cavaillon, JM. Septic shock. *Lancet* 2005;365:63-78.
[18] 18.Vincent JL. Dear SIRS, I'm sorry to say that I don't like you. *Crit. Care Med.* 1997;25:372-374.
[19] Levy MM, Fink MP, Marshall JC, et al. 2001 SCCM/ESICM/ACCP/ATS/SIS international sepsis definitions conference. *Intensive Care Med.* 2003;29:530-538.
[20] Dellinger RP, Levy MM, Carlet JM, et al. Surviving Sepsis Campaign: international guidelines for management of severe sepsis and septic shock: 2008. *Intensive Care Med.* 2008;34:17-60.
[21] Marshall JC, Cook DJ, Christou NV, et al. Multiple organ dysfunction score: a reliable descriptor of a complex clinical outcome. *Crit. Care Med.* 1995;23:1638-1652.
[22] Beutler B. Inferences, questions and possibilities in toll-like receptor signalling. *Nature.* 2004;430:257-263.
[23] Aird WC. The role of the endothelium in severe sepsis and multiple organ dysfunction syndrome. *Blood.* 2003;101:3765-3777.
[24] Brun-Buisson C, Doyon F, Carlet J, et al. Incidence, risk factors, and outcome of severe sepsis and septic shock in adults: a multicenter prospective study in intensive care units: French ICU Group for Severe Sepsis. *JAMA.* 1995;274:968-974.
[25] Estenssoro E, Gonzalez F, Laffaire E, et al. Shock on admission day is the best predictor of prolonged mechanical ventilation in the ICU. *Chest* 2005;127:598-603.
[26] Rackow EC, Astiz ME. Pathophysiology and treatment of septic shock. *JAMA.* 1991;266:548-554.
[27] Karimova A, Pinsky DJ. The endothelial response to oxygen deprivation: biology and clinical implications. *Intensive Care Med.* 2001;27:19-31.
[28] Ogawa S, Koga S, Kuwabara K, et al. Hypoxia-induced increased permeability of endothelial monolayers occurs through lowering of cellular cAMP levels. *Am. J. Physiol.* 1992;262:C546-554.
[29] Shreeniwas R, Koga S, Karakurum M, et al. Hypoxia-mediated induction of endothelial cell interleukin-1 alpha: an autocrine mechanism promoting expression of leukocyte adhesion molecules on the vessel surface. *J. Clin. Invest.* 1992;90:2333-2339.

[30] Lawson CA, Yan SD, Yan SF, et al. Monocytes and tissue factor promote thrombosis in a murine model of oxygen deprivation. *J. Clin. Invest.* 1997;99:1729-1738.

[31] Erickson LA, Fici GJ, Lund JE, et al. Development of venous occlusions in mice transgenic for the plasminogen activator inhibitor-1 gene. *Nature.* 1990;346:74-76.

[32] Astiz ME, Rackow EC, Kaufman B, et al. Relationship of oxygen delivery and mixed venous oxygenation to lactic acidosis in patients with sepsis and acute myocardial infarction. *Crit. Care Med.* 1988;16:655-658.

[33] Parrillo JE, Burch C, Shelhamer JH, et al. A circulating myocardial depressant substance in humans with septic shock: septic shock patients with a reduced ejection fraction have a circulating factor that depresses in vitro myocardial cell performance. *J. Clin. Invest.* 1985;76:1539-1553.

[34] Rivers EP, Ander DS, Powell D. Central venous oxygen saturation monitoring in the critically ill patient. *Curr. Opin. Crit. Care.* 2001;7:204-211.

[35] Scheinman MM, Brown MA, Rapaport E. Critical assessment of use of central venous oxygen saturation as a mirror of mixed venous oxygen in severely ill cardiac patients. *Circulation.* 1969;40:165-172.

[36] Reinhart K, Kuhn HJ, Hartog C, et al. Continuous central venous and pulmonary artery oxygen saturation monitoring in the critically ill. *Intensive Care Med.* 2004;30:1572-1578.

[37] Reinhart K, Rudolph T, Bredle DL, et al. Comparison of central-venous to mixed-venous oxygen saturation during changes in oxygen supply/demand. *Chest.* 1989;95:1216-1221.

[38] Goldman RH, Klughaupt M, Metcalf T, et al. Measurement of central venous oxygen saturation in patients with myocardial infarction. *Circulation.* 1968;38:941-946.

[39] Berridge JC. Influence of cardiac output on the correlation between mixed venous and central venous oxygen saturation. *Br. J. Anaesth.* 1992;69:409-410.

[40] Edwards JD, Mayall RM. Importance of the sampling site for measurement of mixed venous oxygen saturation in shock. *Crit. Care Med.* 1998;26:1356-1360.

[41] Lee J, Wright F, Barber R, et al. Central venous oxygen saturation in shock: a study in man. *Anesthesiology.* 1972;36:472-478.

[42] Scalea TM, Holman M, Fuortes M, et al. Central venous blood oxygen saturation: an early, accurate measurement of volume during hemorrhage. *J. Trauma.* 1988;28:725-732.

[43] Chawla LS, Zia H, Gutierrez G, et al. Lack of equivalence between central and mixed venous oxygen saturation. *Chest.* 2004;126:1891-1896.

[44] Bernardin G, Pradier C, Tiger F, et al. Blood pressure and arterial lactate level are early indicators of short-term survival in human septic shock. *Intensive Care Med.* 1996;22:17-25.

[45] Wo CC, Shoemaker WC, Appel PL, et al. Unreliability of blood pressure and hart rate to evaluate cardiac output in emergency resuscitation and critical illness. *Crit. Care Med.* 1993;21:218-223.

[46] Rady M, Rivers EP, Nowak RM. Resuscitation of the critically ill in the ED: responses of blood pressure, heart rate, shock index, central venous saturation, and lactate. *Am. J. Emerg Med.* 1996;2:218-225.

[47] Fink MP. Cytopathic hypoxia: mitochondrial dysfunction as mechanism contributing to organ dysfunction in sepsis. *Crit. Care Clin.* 2001; 17:219-237.

[48] Fink MP. Cytopathic hypoxia: is oxygen use impaired in sepsis as a result of an acquired intrinsic derangement in cellular respiration? *Crit. Care Clin.* 2002;18:165-175.

[49] Nguyen HB, Rivers EP, Abrahamian FM, et al. Severe Sepsis and Septic Shock: Review of the Literature and Emergency Department Management Guidelines. *Ann. Emerg. Med.* 2006;48:28-54.

[50] Norman DC, Yoshikawa TT. Fever in the elderly. *Infect Dis Clin North Am.* 1996;10:93-99.

[51] Chassagne P, Perol MB, Doucet J, et al. Is presentation of bacteremia in the elderly the same as in younger patients? *Am. J. Med.* 1996;100:65-70.

[52] Morris DL, Chambers HF, Morris MG, et al. Hemodynamic characteristics of patients with hypothermia due to occult infection and other causes. *Ann. Intern Med.* 1985;102:153-157.

[53] Cornbleet PJ. Clinical utility of the band count. *Clin. Lab. Med.* 2002;22:101-136.

[54] Novak RW. The beleaguered band count. *Clin. Lab. Med.* 1993; 13:895-903.

[55] Wenz B, Gennis P, Canova C, et al. The clinical utility of the leukocyte differential in emergency medicine. *Am. J. Clin. Pathol.*1986;86:298-303.

[56] Ardron MJ, Westengard JC, Dutcher TF. Band neutrophil counts are unnecessary for the diagnosis of infection in patients with normal total leukocyte counts. *Am. J. Clin. Pathol.* 1994;102:646-649.
[57] Callaham M. Inaccuracy and expense of the leukocyte count in making urgent clinical decisions. *Ann. Emerg. Med.* 1986;15:774-781.
[58] Kuppermann N, Walton EA. Immature neutrophils in the blood smears of young febrile children. *Arch. Pediatr. Adolesc. Med.*1999;153:261-266.
[59] Vanderschueren S, De Weerdt A, Malbrain M, et al. Thrombocytopenia and prognosis in intensive care. *Crit. Care Med.* 2000;28:1871-1876.
[60] Powars D, Larsen R, Johnson J, et al. Epidemic meningococcemia and purpura fulminans with induced protein C deficiency. *Clin. Infect Dis.* 1993;17:254-261.
[61] Fourrier F, Chopin C, Goudemand J, et al. Septic shock, multiple organ failure, and disseminated intravascular coagulation: compared patterns of antithrombin III, protein C, and protein S deficiencies. *Chest.* 1992;101:816-823.
[62] Levraut J, Bounatirou T, Ichai C, et al. Reliability of anion gap as an indicator of blood lactate in critically ill patients. *Intensive Care Med.* 1997;23:417-422.
[63] Iberti TJ, Leibowitz AB, Papadakos PJ, et al. Low sensitivity of the anion gap as a screen to detect hyperlactatemia in critically ill patients. *Crit. Care Med.* 1990;18:275-277.
[64] Abramson D, Scalea TM, Hitchcock R, et al. Lactate clearance and survival following injury. *J. Trauma.* 1993;35:584-588.
[65] Bakker J, Gris P, Coffernils M, et al. Serial blood lactate levels can predict the development of multiple organ failure following septic shock. *Am. J. Surg.* 1996;171:221-226.
[66] Shapiro NI, Howell MD, Talmor D, et al. Serum lactate as a predictor of mortality in emergency department patients with infection. *Ann. Emerg. Med.* 2005;45:524-528.
[67] Nguyen HB, Rivers EP, Knoblich BP, et al. Early lactate clearance is associated with improved outcome in severe sepsis and septic shock. *Crit. Care Med.* 2004;32:1637-1642.
[68] Miguel BV, Casanoves LEB, Pallas BL, et al. Prognostic value of the biomarkers procalcitonin, interleukin-6 and C-reactive protein in severe sepsis. *Med. Intensiva.*2012
[69] Marshall JC, Vincent JL, Fink MP, et al. Measures, markers, and mediators: toward a staging system for clinical sepsis: a report of the

Fifth Toronto Sepsis Roundtable, Toronto, Ontario,Canada, October 25-26, 2000. *Crit. Care Med.* 2003;31:1560-1567.

[70] Gibot S, Kolopp-Sarda MN, BénéMC, et al. Plasma level of a triggering receptor expressed on myeloid cells-1: its diagnostic accuracy in patients with suspected sepsis. *Ann. Intern. Med.* 2004;141:9-15.

[71] Gibot S, Cravoisy A, Kolopp-Sarda MN, et al. Time-course of sTREM (soluble triggering receptor expressed on myeloid cells)-1, procalcitonin, and C-reactive protein plasma concentrations during sepsis. *Crit. Care Med.* 2005;33:792-796.

[72] Gibot S, Le Renard PE, Bollaert PE, et al. Surface triggering receptor expressed on myeloid cells 1 expression patterns in septic shock. *Intensive Care Med.* 2005;31:594-597.

[73] Mandell LA, Bartlett JG, Dowell SF, et al. Update of practice guidelines for the management of community-acquired pneumonia in immunocompetent adults. *Clin. Infect Dis.* 2003; 37:1405-1433.

[74] Boissinot M, Bergeron MG. Toward rapid real-time molecular diagnostic to guide smart use of antimicrobials. *Curr. Opin. Microbiol.* 2002;5:478-482.

[75] Sessler CN, Perry JC, Varney KL. Management of severe sepsis and septic shock. *Curr. Opin. Crit. Care.* 2004;10:354-363.

[76] Luce JM. Pathogenesis and management of septic shock. *Chest.* 1987;91:883-888.

[77] Ghosh S, Latimer RD, Gray BM, et al. Endotoxin-induced organ injury. *Crit. Care Med.* 1993;21:S19-S24.

[78] Michard F, Boussat S, Chemla D, et al. Relation between respiratory changes in arterial pulse pressure and fluid responsiveness in septic patients with acute circulatory failure. *Am. J. Respir. Crit. Care Med* 2000;162:134-138.

[79] Walley KR. Use of central venous oxygen saturation to guide therapy. *Am. J. Respir. Crit. Care Med* 2011;184:514-520.

[80] Harvey S, Harrison DA, Singer M, et al. Assessment of the clinical effectiveness of pulmonary artery catheters in management of patients in intensive care (PAC-Man): a randomised controlled trial. *Lancet* 2005; 366:472-477.

[81] National Heart, Lung, and Blood Institute Acute Respiratory Distress Syndrome (ARDS) Clinical Trials Network, Wheeler AP, Bernard GR, et al. Pulmonary-artery versus central venous catheter to guide treatment of acute lung injury. *N. Engl. J. Med.* 2006; 354:2213-2224.

[82] Jones AE, Shapiro NI, Trzeciak S, et al. Lactate clearance vs central venous oxygen saturation as goals of early sepsis therapy: a randomized clinical trial. *JAMA* 2010; 303:739-746.
[83] Forsythe SM, Schmidt GA. Sodium bicarbonate for the treatment of lactic acidosis. *Chest* 2000; 117:260-267.
[84] 84.Gutierrez G, Palizas F, Doglio G, et al. Gastric intramucosal pH as a therapeutic index of tissue oxygenation in critically ill patients. *Lancet* 1992; 339:195-199.
[85] Poeze M, Solberg BC, Greve JW, et al. Monitoring global volume-related hemodynamic or regional variables after initial resuscitation: What is a better predictor of outcome in critically ill septic patients? *Crit. Care Med.* 2005; 33:2494-2500.
[86] Wheeler AP, Bernard GR. Treating patients with severe sepsis. *N. Engl. J. Med.* 1999; 340:207-.214.
[87] Presiser JC, Devos P, Ruiz-Santana S, et al. A prospective randomised multicentre controlled trial on the tight glycemic control by intensive insulin therapy in adult intensive care units: the Glucontrol study. *Intensive Care Med.* 2009;35:1738-1748.
[88] Brunkhorst FM, Engel C, Bloos F, et al. Intensive insulin therapy and pentastarch resuscitation in severe sepsis. *N. Eng. J. Med.* 2008;358:125-39.
[89] Finfer S, Chittock DR, SuSY, et al. Intensive versus conventional glucose control in critically ill patients. *N. Eng. J. Med.* 2009;360:1283-1297.
[90] Martí-Carvajal AJ, Solà I, Lathyris D, Cardona AF. Human recombinant activated protein C for severe sepsis. *Cochrane Database Syst. Rev.* 2012;3:CD004388.
[91] Gaieski DF, Mikkelsen ME, Band RA, et al. Impact of time to antibiotics on survival in patients with severe sepsis or septic shock in whom early goal-directed therapy was initiated in the emergency department. *Crit. Care Med* 2010;38:1045-1053.
[92] Johnson MT, Reichley R, Hoppe-Bauer J, et al. Impact of previous antibiotic therapy on outcome of Gram-negative severe sepsis. *Crit. Care Med.* 2011;39:1859-1865.
[93] Verhoef J, Hustinx WM, Frasa H, et al. Issues in the adjunct therapy of severe sepsis. *J. Antimicrob. Chemother* 1996;38:167-182.
[94] Sibbald WJ, Vincent JL. Round table conference on clinical trials for the treatment of sepsis. *Crit. Care Med.* 1995;23:394-399.

[95] Garnacho-Montero J, Garcia-Garmendia JL, Barrero-Almodovar A, et al. Impact of adequate empirical antibiotic therapy on the outcome of patients admitted to the intensive care unit with sepsis. *Crit. Care Med.* 2003;31:2742-2751.

[96] Ibrahim EH, Sherman G, Ward S, et al. The influence of inadequate antimicrobial treatment of bloodstream infections on patient outcomes in the ICU setting. *Chest* 2000;118:146-155.

[97] Harbarth S, Garbino J, Pugin J, et al. Inappropriate initial antimicrobial therapy and its effect on survival in a clinical trial of immunomodulating therapy for severe sepsis. *Am. J. Med.* 2003;115:529-535.

[98] Leibovici L, Paul M, Poznanski O, et al. Monotherapy versus beta-lactam-aminoglycoside combination treatment for gram-negative bacteremia: a prospective, observational study. *Antimicrob. Agents Chemother.* 1997; 41:1127-1133.

[99] Kumar A, Roberts D, Wood KE, et al. Duration of hypotension before initiation of effective antimicrobial therapy is the critical determinant of survival in human septic shock. *Crit. Care Med.* 2006; 34:1589-1596.

[100] Schramm GE, Johnson JA, Doherty JA, et al. Methicillin-resistant Staphylococcus aureus sterile-site infection: The importance of appropriate initial antimicrobial treatment. *Crit. Care Med.* 2006; 34:2069-2074.

[101] Kumar A, Ellis P, Arabi Y, et al. Initiation of inappropriate antimicrobial therapy results in a fivefold reduction of survival in human septic shock. *Chest* 2009; 136:1237.

[102] McDonald JR, Friedman ND, Stout JE, et al. Risk factors for ineffective therapy in patients with bloodstream infection. *Arch. Intern. Med.* 2005;165:308-313.

[103] Annane D, Sebille V, Charpentier C, et al. Effect of treatment with low doses of hydrocortisone and fludrocortisone on mortality in patients with septic shock. *JAMA* 2002; 288:862-871.

[104] Sprung CL, Annane D, Keh D, et al. Hydrocortisone therapy for patients with septic shock. *N. Eng. J. Med.* 2008; 358:111-124.

[105] Heyland DK, Dhaliwal R, Drover JW, et al. Canadian clinical practice guidelines for nutrition support in mechanically ventilated, critically ill adult patients. *JPEN J. Parenter Enteral Nutr.* 2003; 27:355-373.

[106] Kondrup J, Allison SP, Elia M, et al. ESPEN guidelines for nutrition screening 2002. *Clin Nutr* 2003; 22:415-421.

[107] Ziegler TR. Nutrition support in critical illness—bridging the evidence gap. *N. Eng. J. Med.* 2011; 365: 506-517.

[108] Seres DS. Surrogate nutrition markers, malnutrition, and adequancy of nutrition support. *Nutr. Clin. Pract.* 2005; 20:308-313.
[109] Heyland DK, Cahill N, Day AG. Optimal amount of calories for critically ill patients: depends on how you slice the cake! *Crit. Care Med.* 2011; 39:2619-2626.
[110] Artinian V, Krayem H, DiGiovine B. Effects of early enteral feeding on the outcome of critically ill mechanically ventilated medical patients. *Chest* 2006; 129:960-967.
[111] Marik PE, Zaloga GP. Early enteral nutrition in acutely ill patients: a systematic review. *Crit. Care Med.* 2001; 29:2264-2270.
[112] Koretz RL, Avenell A, Lipman TO, et al. Does enteral nutrition affect clinical outcome? A systematic review of the randomized trials. *Am. J. Gastroenterol.* 2007;102:412-429.
[113] Casaer MP, Mesotten D, Hermans G, et al. Early versus late parenteral nutrition in critically ill adults. *N. Engl. J. Med.* 2011; 365:506-517.
[114] Dvir D, Cohen J, Singer P. Computerized energy balance and complications in critically ill patients: an observational study. *Clin. Nutr.* 2006; 25:37-44.
[115] Kortgen A, Niederprüm P, Bauer M. Implementation of an evidence-based "standard operating procedure" and outcome in septic shock. *Crit. Care Med.* 2006;34:943-949.
[116] Shapiro NI, Howell MD, Talmor D, et al. Implementation and outcomes of the Multiple Urgent Sepsis Therapies (MUST) protocol. *Crit. Care Med.* 2006;34:1025-1032.
[117] Micek ST, Roubinian N, Heuring T, et al. Before-after study of a standardized hospital order set for the management of septic shock. *Crit. Care Med.* 2006;34:2707-2713.
[118] Schramm GE, Kashyap R, Mullon JJ, Gajic O, Afessa B. Septic shock: a multidisciplinary response team and weekly feedback to clinicians improve the process of care and mortality. *Crit. Care Med.* 2011;39:252-258.

In: Septic Shock
Editors: M. Johnston and J. Knight

ISBN: 978-1-62257-485-8
© 2012 Nova Science Publishers, Inc.

Chapter 3

SEPTIC SHOCK:
CLINICAL DIAGNOSIS AND RISK FACTORS

Diego Saa, Fernanda Galleguillos,
Catherine Céspedes and Ramón Rodrigo[*]
Renal Pathophysiology Laboratory,
Molecular and Clinical Pharmacology Program,
Institute of Biomedical Sciences, Faculty of Medicine,
University of Chile, Santiago, Chile

ABSTRACT

Septic shock is an important cause of mortality among critically ill patients. It arises out of a complex interaction between a susceptible host and a virulent pathogen. This interaction causes a massive release of different inflammatory mediators, reactive oxygen and nitrogen species and microbial antigens to bloodstream, and activation of different cell populations, e.g. leukocytes and endothelial cells. The result of such chaotic, uncontrolled and deregulated inflammatory cascade damages different organ tissues, which leads to multiple organ dysfunction syndrome and eventually, death. Once diagnosed the occurrence of septic shock, antibiotic and fluid therapies have been proven effective, while

---

[*] Corresponding author: Dr. Ramón Rodrigo, Molecular and Clinical Pharmacology Program, Institute of Biomedical Sciences, Faculty of Medicine, University of Chile. Email: rrodrigo@med.uchile.cl, Address: Reyes Lavalle 3415, Depto. 71, Las Condes, C.P 7550164, Santiago, Región Metropolitana, Chile

identification of this condition remains challenging. So, to increase survival rates and to improve clinical outcomes in critically ill patients, clinical behavior should be focused in early and accurate identification of risk factors and diagnosis. Also novel biomarkers research and development of new diagnostic laboratory tools should be promoted. Altogether, these progresses may provide a better understanding of the pathophysiological mechanisms underlying this pathology, which could result in better and earlier target-specific therapeutical strategies to prevent its progression to multiple organ dysfunction syndrome and death.

Keywords: Inflammation – SIRS – Sepsis – Shock – MODS

ABBREVIATIONS

ABG	Arterial blood gases
ACCP	American College of Chest Physicians
AP-1	Activator protein-1
APACHE score	Acute physiology and chronic health evaluation
aPTT	Activated partial tromboplastin time
ATS	American Thoracic Society
BE	Base excess
BP	Blood pressure
BUN	Blood urea nitrogen
CARS	Compensatory anti-inflammatory response syndrome
Casp-3	Caspase 3
CAT	Catalase
CBC	Complete blood count
CRP	C-reactive protein
DIC	Disseminated intravascular coagulation
EMS	Emergency medical services
ER	Emergency department
ESICM	European Society of Intensive Care Medicine
FDP	Fibrin degradation products
GCS	Glasgow coma scale
GPx	Glutathione peroxidase
GSH	Glutathione
HF	Hospital floor
HIV	Human immunodeficiency virus

ICAM-1	Intercellular adhesion molecule-1
ICU	Intensive care unit
IL-1, -1β -6, -8, -18	Interleukin-1, -1 β, -6, -8, -18
IL-1Ra	Interleukin-1 receptor antagonist
INR	International normalized ratio
MAP	Mean arterial pressure
MDA	Malondialdehyde
MODS	Multiple organ dysfunction syndrome
MPO	Mieloperoxidase
MV	Mechanical ventilation
NADPH	Reduced Nicotine adenine dinucleotide phosphate
NF-κB	Nuclear factor kappa-light chain enhancer of activated B cells
NIH	National Institutes of Health
NK cells	Natural killer cells
NO	Nitric oxide
PCT	Procalcitonin
PICU	Pediatric intensive care unit
PT	Protrombin time
RNA	Ribonucleic acid
ROC curve	Receiver operating characteristic curve
RONS	Reactive oxygen and nitrogen species
ROS	Reactive oxygen species
SBP	Systolic blood pressure
SCCM	Society of Critical Care Medicine
ScvO$_2$	Mixed venous oxygen saturation
Sel-P	Selenoprotein-P
SH-groups	Thiol groups
SIRS	Systemic inflammatory response syndrome
SIS	Surgical Infection Society
SOAP study	The Sepsis Occurrence in Acutely ill Patients study
SOD	Superoxide dismutase
SOFA score	Sequential Organ Failure Assessment
SSC	Surviving Sepsis Campaign
TBARS	Thiobarbituric acid reactant substances
TNF-α	Tumor necrosis factor-α
WBC	White blood cell
XO	Xanthine oxidase

1. Introduction

1.1. Basic Concepts

Early in the 1990's decade a Consensus Conference hosted by the American College of Chest Physicians (ACCP) and the Society of Critical Care Medicine (SCCM) established definitions for adult septic patients [1].

This conference represents a turning point as it provides a common language for research in sepsis, defining key concepts (see Table 1) [1,2] and establishing guidelines for the use of innovative therapies.

Finally it also recommended eliminating the old term "septicaemia", since it straddles the definitions of sepsis, severe sepsis, and septic shock [1,3]. To date, these definitions remain largely accepted and unchanged.

Furthermore, different scientific societies such as the European Society of Intensive Care Medicine (ESICM), the American Thoracic Society (ATS) and the Surgical Infection Society (SIS) have validated them, ratified its use in clinical settings and complemented them in a International Conference [2]. The complements to the initial definitions have been summarized in Table 1.

Finally, it is noteworthy that despite the efforts to generalize these definitions to the pediatric population, special characteristics of these patients have to be taken under consideration; hence diagnostic criteria differ from those used in adults as defined in 2005 by the International Consensus Conference on Pediatric Sepsis [4].

1.2. Epidemiological Impact of Sepsis and Septic Shock

The sepsis syndrome consists in a wide spectrum of conditions that have become an important health care issue, because of its increasing incidence, morbidity, mortality and costs associated. In large epidemiological studies of up to 6 million people an incidence of 3 per 1000 population per year or about 750000 cases a year in the United States was determined [3], but this number could be underestimated due to low diagnostic rate and accuracy or difficulties in tracking sepsis in many countries [5]. Thus, the importance of sepsis is increasing year by year and it is thought to affect 18 million patients each year [5,6]. Noteworthy is that mortality has been decreasing, even though it remains unacceptably high [6–8].

Similarly, in Europe a observational, prospective and multicentre study - The SOAP Study- showed marked differences in the frequency of sepsis between countries, and higher frequencies of sepsis were correlated with higher mortality rates [7,9].

In addition, assessment of key organ systems shows that increasing severity of organ dysfunction and the number of involved organ systems correlates with increasing mortality, which rises from 25-30% for severe sepsis up to 40-70% for septic shock in adults [3]. This has also been ratified by the SOAP study, where patients with no organ dysfunction on admission had mortality rates of 6%, in comparison to those with four or more organ failures whose mortality rates were 65% [9–11].

Increasing incidence can be explained in terms of numerous contributing factors, ie. aging patients, immunosuppression due to aggressive cancer therapy or to increased prevalence of HIV, and multidrug-resistant infections due to indiscriminate use of broad spectrum antibiotics [7,8]. Furthermore, it has been found that comorbidities influence the risk and outcome of sepsis and those cumulative comorbidities are associated with greater organ dysfunction [8].

On the other hand, decreasing mortality has been attributed to earlier and general improvements in acute and intensive hospital care, rather to better understanding of sepsis pathophysiology or to targeted-specific interventions directed to prevent the development and persistence of multiple organ dysfunction syndrome (MODS), the major contributor to death in most instances [8].

Finally, sepsis-associated costs account for a huge impact on hospitals' finances, since critical care units consume large amounts of resources, and are target for reducing medical expenses. In USA, caring for a septic patient on average demands approximately US$22,000, corresponding to US$16.7 billion each year. These figures may increase, as severity of disease progresses to severe sepsis, septic shock or MODS. Thus, when compared, the cost of treating an ICU patient with sepsis has been shown to be 6-fold higher than that of treating a patient without sepsis [5,12].

In addition, social impact of sepsis results from productivity loss due to absenteeism, sequelae or mortality. Thus, these indirect costs have been estimated to be as high as 2-3 times the direct costs.

For these reasons, healthcare providers, managers, government authorities, and insurance companies have focused their attention on strategies that could reduce the economic and social burden of sepsis [12].

Table 1. Definitions of the ACCP/SCCM Consensus Conference Committee [1], complements by the SCCM/ESICM/ACCP/ATS/SIS International Sepsis Definitions Conference [2] and pediatric criteria by the Internacional pediatric sepsis consensus conference [4]

Concept	Definition	Diagnostic Criteria or Parameters
Systemic inflammatory response syndrome (SIRS)	Unspecific and stereotyped systemic inflammatory response to a variety of severe insults.	Two or more of the following: (a) Core temperature > 38°C or < 36°. (b) Heart rate (HR) > 90 bpm or > 2 SD for age or in children <1 year: HR < p10 (c) Respiratory rate (RR) >20 breaths/min or $PaCO_2$ < 32 mm Hg, or RR > 2SD for age or acute mechanical ventilation need in absence of neuromuscular disease or anesthetics. (d) White blood cell count >12,000/cu mm, <4000/cu mm or >10% immature (bands) forms. *In children, two or more of these criteria must be fulfilled and at least either core temperature or altered WBC count must be one of them.*
Sepsis	Systemic inflammatory response as a result of a confirmed or suspected infection.	1. General: (a) Previous SIRS parameters: Fever or Hypothermia, Tachycardia and Tachypnea. (b) Significant edema or positive fluid balance (>20 ml/kg over 24 h). (c) Hyperglycemia (plasma glucose >110 mg/dl or 7.7 mM/l) in the absence of diabetes 2. Inflammation: (a) Previous SIRS parameters: Leukocitosis, Leukopenia or Normal WBC count with >10% immature foms. (b) Plasma C reactive protein (CRP) >2 SD above the normal value. (b) Plasma procalcitonin (PCT) >2 SD above the normal value.
Severe sepsis	Sepsis associated with organ dysfunction, hypoperfusion or hypotension (ie. Lactic acidosis, oliguria, acute mental status alteration).	1. Hemodinamic criteria (a) Arterial hypotension: Systolic blood pressure (SBP) <90 mmHg, Mean arterial pressure (MAP) <70, or a SBP decrease >40 mmHg in adults. (b) Mixed venous oxygen saturation ($ScvO_2$) >70% (c) Cardiac index >3.5 l/min/m^2.

In children, after administration of isotonic fluid bolus 40 ml/kg/h:

(a) Hypotension < p5 for age or SBP < 2 SD for age, or
(b) Vasoactive drug to maintain a normal BP (dopamin > 5 μg/kg/min, dobutamine, epinephrine o norepinephrine in any dose), or
(c) Two of the following: Unexplained metabolic acidosis (BE < -5.0 mEq/l); Elevated arterial lactate > 2 normal value; Oliguria (urine output < 0.5 ml/kg/h), capillary refill > 5 s, core/peripheral temperature difference > 3°C

In children corresponds to sepsis associated with cardiovascular disfunction or acute respiratory distress syndrome (ARDS), or 2 or more organ dysfunctions.

2. Organ dysfunction
(a) Respiratory dysfunction: Arterial hypoxemia (PaO_2/F_iO_2 <300)
(i) In children: PaO_2/F_iO_2 < 300 in absence of preexisting cianotic cheart or pulmonary disease; or $PaCO_2$ > 65 torr or 20 mm Hg above baseline pCO_2; increases in O_2 requirements or F_iO_2 > 50% to maintain $SatO_2$ 92%; or need for invasive or non-invasive mechanical ventilation.
(b) Renal dysfunction: Acute oliguria (urine output <0.5 ml/kg/h or 45 mM/l for at least 2 h) or Creatinine increase ≥0.5 mg/dl
(i) In children: Serum creatinine > 2 times normal value for age or > 2 times baseline value.
(c) Hematologic dysfunction: Thrombocytopenia (platelet count <100,000/μl)
(i) In children: Platelets < 80.000/mm; or 50% decrease in last count over the last 3 days (in chronic hemato-oncologic patients); or INR > 2.
(d) Liver dysfunction: Hyperbilirubinemia (plasma total bilirubin >4 mg/dl or 70 mmol/l); Coagulation abnormalities (INR >1.5 or aPTT >60 s)
(i) In children: Total bilirrubin > 4 mg/dl (not for newborn); or Alanine transaminase 2 times normal value for age.
(e) Gastrointestina dysfunction: Ileus (absent bowel sounds)
(f) In children: Neurologic dysfunction: Glasgow coma scale (GCS) < 11; or acute mental status alteration with 3 points decrease in baseline GCS.

3. Tissue hypoperfusion
(a) Hyperlactacidemia (>3 mmol/l)
(b) Decreased capillary refill or mottling

Sepsis-induced hypotension	Systolic blood pressure of < 90 mm Hg or a decrease of > 40 mm Hg from baseline, in absence of other causes of hypotension.

Table 1. (Continued)

Concept	Definition	Diagnostic Criteria or Parameters
Sepsis-induced hypotension	Systolic blood pressure of < 90 mm Hg or a decrease of > 40 mm Hg from baseline, in absence of other causes of hypotension.	
Septic shock	Sepsis-induced hypotension despite adequate fluid resuscitation along with perfusion abnormalities (ie. Lactic acidosis, oliguria, acute mental status alteration).	
	In children, sepsis with cardiovascular dysfunction.	
Multiple organ dysfunction syndrome (MODS)	Presence of altered organ functions in an acutely ill patient, such that homeostasis cannot be maintained without intervention.	

Table 2. Suggested clinical approach to the septic patient in the ER

Clinical assessment	Suggested actions	Suggested evaluations
1. Identification of life-threatening signs	Evaluate for hemodynamic instability, peripheral hypoperfusion, respiratory distress, petechiae, meningeal signs, acute abdomen and severe hyperthermia	
2. History	Collect personal history and family information regarding overall health, presence of comorbidities and control level, and symptoms suggesting infections.	Consider contact with other patients diagnosed and treated for severe contagious diseases (eg. Meningococcemia)
3. Physical Examination	Comprehensive, systematical and repeated assessment of worsening general conditions and identification of possible septic sources.	
4. Diagnosis	Early diagnosis should lead to sepsis-specific protocol enrollment, so that both diagnoses can promptly be confirmed and adequate therapy initiated.	
5. Infectious source identification	Clinically suspected sources should be confirmed by all means necessary. If no clear source is identified, repeated assessment should be performed to identify other overlooked sources.	The most common sites of infection are lung (35%), abdomen (21%), urinary tract (13%), skin and soft tissue (7%), other site (8%), and unknown primary site (16%) [20].
6. Additional tests	Basic laboratory tests in order to evaluate baseline status assess clinical response to therapy and to determine organ dysfunction. Additionally, imagenologic studies aimed to identify specific sources when no clear source has been initially recognized.	CBC analysis with the differential and Eritrosedimentation rate (ESR) Arterial blood gas (ABG), serum electrolytes and lactate. Blood chemistry, serum glucose, serum billirrubin and liver enzymes, protrombin time (PT) and INR, activated partial trombloplastin time (aPTT). Serum creatinine, blood uric nitrogen (BUN) and Urinalysis.

2. CLINICAL APPROACH TO THE SEPTIC PATIENT

As outlined by the "Barcelona Declaration" in October 2002, the Surviving Sepsis Campaign (SSC) has called for action against sepsis, in order to secure the support of governments, health care agencies and professionals to help lower the relative mortality of sepsis by 25% over the next 5 years. Considering that early treatment is associated to better outcomes, the objective of the SSC is to raise awareness of the challenges associated with sepsis. The fundamental challenge is the difficulty in its diagnosis, because no consensus on the clinical definition of sepsis exists [5]. Therefore, this chapter addresses this essential issue, with emphasis on the diagnostic biomarkers currently used in clinical settings and newly developed biomarkers under active research.

2.1. Suspected Sepsis in the ER

Pathophysiologically, sepsis develops as a result of the inflammatory response of the host to an infectious insult. Considering the magnitude of the septic insult and the intensity of the corresponding inflammatory response of the host, it can progress from a localized, well-circumscribed and time-limited process to a systemic and life-threatening condition that can lead to multiple organ dysfunction, and eventually death. Finally, it also has to be taken into account that later on the course of sepsis, patients also present with immunosuppressive features thanks to the compensatory anti-inflammatory response syndrome (CARS) [13], including: loss of delayed hypersensitivity, the difficulty or impossibility in some cases to eliminate autonomously the source of infection, and susceptibility to nosocomial infections [14].

Thus, clinical manifestations are widely variable according to severity. Clinical severity, as previously stated is influenced by several factors, ie. etiology, site of infection, clinical interventions and host factors, such as: genetics, baseline health and presence of comorbidities. So, clinical findings are varied and may be so subtle that a high level of diagnostic suspicion is required. In presence of sepsis-suspected patients in the Emergency Department (ER), clinical judgment should be complemented with appropriate laboratory tests in an effort to distinguish sepsis from non-infectious SIRS and initiating early, timely and effective therapeutical interventions.

Early recognition of sepsis is important because of the morbidity and mortality associated. Wang et al. demonstrated in a study conducted in China that patients who develop septic shock in the ER compared to those do on

Hospital Floors (HF) have lower in-hospital mortality, less use of mechanical ventilation (MV) during the first 24 hours following onset of septic shock and the HF patients required a longer time to achieve target $ScvO_2$. The need for mechanical ventilation was independently associated with increased mortality [15]. Finally, Band et al. demonstrated that arriving by emergency medical services (EMS) was was associated with improved in-hospital processes for the care of critically ill patients, shortening ER treatment times for septic patients, although a mortality benefit could not be demonstrated [16].

A fully detailed algorithm about the clinical approach to the septic patient in the ER is presented on Table 2.

2.2. Patients at Risk of Septic Shock

As important as early recognition of septic patients for on-time therapy initiation, is the identification of several risk factors that could help predict those patients who will develop a more severe disease. In this line of thought, Rangel-Fausto et al. in 1998 using Markov models in a prospective cohort study in three different ICU and three general wards in tertiary health institutions estimated the probability of movement to and from different stages of the SIRS-sepsis spectrum of disease. In general, the probability of patients on day 1 to stay in the same stage of disease –either sepsis, severe sepsis or septic shock- was 65%, 68% and 61%, respectively; while the probability of progression from sepsis to severe sepsis was 9% and from severe sepsis to septic shock was 2.6%. Finally, probability of dying in patients with sepsis, severe sepsis and septic shock was 0.5%, 0.9% and 7.9%, respectively [17].

However, data regarding specific risk factors for worsening sepsis in infected patients was still lacking. In 2005, Alberti et al. designed a study focused on determining clinical variables associated with worsening sepsis. In this study, they found that approximately one of four patients presenting with infection/sepsis developed severe sepsis or shock, and variables independently associated with progression were: temperature over 38.2ºC; heart rate over 120/minute, systolic blood pressure higher than 110 mmHg, platelets higher than 150.000 /dL, serum sodium over 145 mmol/L, bilirubin over 30 umol/L, mechanical ventilation, and infection-characterizing variables (pneumonia, peritonitis, primary bacteremia, and infection with gram-positive cocci or aerobic gram-negative bacilli). In addition, a score was developed with these variables to stratify patients in risk categories of progressing to severe sepsis or septic shock [18].

2.3. Confirming the Diagnosis

2.3.1. Laboratory Analyses and Work-Up

Once sepsis diagnosis is suspected, prompt confirmation is required for instauration of adequate therapeutic actions. A comprehensive laboratory evaluation is imperative in order to fulfill 3 important objectives: (a) To fully assess the current clinical status of the patient, establish a clinical health baseline and determining organ dysfunction; (b) To stratify patients into risk groups of severity progression and (c) To determine the exact etiology, localization and antimicrobial sensitivity of the causative pathogen. To accomplish these objectives, we propose the following initial approach:

a. General Laboratory tests. A full CBC analysis with the differential and Eritrosedimentation rate (ESR) looking for typical signs of bacterial infections, such as: leukocytosis or leukopenia, neutrophilia or neutropenia, and bandemia (presence of immature forms of granulocytes in peripheral blood). However, this signs alone have poor sensitivity and specificity in diagnosing bacterial infection, and likelihood increases when complemented with other signs such as: Döhle´s bodies, toxic granulation and vacuoles. Other signs often present in the CBC analysis are hemoconcentration due to fluid leakage of the intravascular into the intersticial space or decreased hematocrit after fluid resuscitation. Special attention should be paid to thrombocytopenia, since heralds the onset of disseminated intravascular coagulation (DIC) and acts as independent predictor of poor outcome and MODS [19,20]. Finally, elevated ESR accounts for elevated synthesis of acute-phase proteins in context of inflammation.

Arterial blood gases (ABG), serum electrolytes and lactate allow us to evaluate the acid-base status of the patient, which may reveal metabolic acidosis and hyperlactacidemia, both indicative of tissue hypoperfusion. Also, elevated lactate and base deficit are independent predictor of mortality among septic cancer patients [21].

A standard blood chemistry containing serum glucose, billirrubin, liver enzymes and also coagulation studies, such as protrombin time (PT) and INR, activated partial tromboplastin time (aPTT) are needed to fully assess liver function, presence of hyperglycemia and complete the evaluation when DIC is suspected, along with D-dimer, fibrin degradation products (FDP) and fibrinogen.

Finally, serum creatinine, blood uric nitrogen (BUN) and Urinalysis are required to assess kidney function [19].

   b. Acute-phase reactants. During sepsis the host-pathogen interaction initiates a proinflammatory molecular cascade, which activates different transcription factors such as NF-κB (Nuclear factor kappa-light chain enhancer of activated B cells) and AP-1 (activator protein-1), which further induce the expression of proinflammatory mediators, such as TNF-α, ICAM-1, IL-8, IL-1Ra and Casp-3 [22]. These proinflammatory biomarkers promote synthesis and secretion of so called acute-phase reactants ie. C reactive protein (CRP) and procalcitonin (PCT), which can be used in clinical setting to confirm presence of an inflammatory process [19]. Further discussion about these biomarkers is presented below.
   c. Septic source. However difficult in the ER, establishing a definitive microbial source in context of severe sepsis/septic shock, identification of the organism and determining its antimicrobial susceptibilities are crucial in subsequent management, because clinical outcome relies also on microbiological factors such as the organism involved [19,23,24]. Thus, infections caused by gram negative organisms tend to be localized in the lung, abdomen, bloodstream and urinary tract, while gram positive sources are skin and/or soft tissues, indwelling intravascular lines, urinary catheters or other prosthetic materials, the respiratory tract and the bloodstream [24]. Therefore, appropriate cultures should be taken before antimicrobial treatment, but also must not delay therapy. At least 2 blood cultures should be obtained, with at least 10 mL each, taken one percutaneously and one through each vascular access device and distributed into aerobic and anaerobic bottles [23], since about 50% of patients with severe sepsis/septic shock have positive blood cultures [19]. Based on clinical scenario other possible sources should be investigated. So urine cultures, Sputum or purulent material from skin and/or soft tissue infections and normally sterile fluids -ie. Joint, cerebrospinal, pleural- should be obtained for gram's stain and culture. Finally, when indwelling intravascular or urinary catheter infection is suspected, catheter removal and tip culture are indicated [19].

Another set of testing shown to be useful and available in clinical practice are urinary testing of pneumococcal and *Legionella* antigens, recommended now for patients being admitted to the ICU, those who have failed outpatient treatment, and those with comorbidities [20].

2.3.2. Imaging Studies

The SSC guidelines recommend imaging studies to be performed as soon as possible, in order to confirm a potential source of infection and allowing content sampling. Thus, imaging studies may identify infectious sources requiring removal of foreign body, abscesses drainage or tissue debridement, in order to maximize the therapy response likelihood. Nevertheless, septic patients may be too unstable to warrant certain invasive diagnostic procedures or transport outside the ICU. So, bedside studies such as ultrasound are the proceedings of choice under these circumstances. Balancing risk and benefit is therefore mandatory in those settings [23].

2.3.3. New Diagnostic Tools and Future Research

The concept of biomarkers was first defined by a special panel at the NIH, as any characteristic that is objectively measured and evaluated as an indicator of normal biological processes, pathogenic processes, or pharmacologic responses to a therapeutic intervention. However, in the daily use, this term is applied to any test performed on some body fluid that provides information not readily obtainable otherwise using current diagnostic modalities [25].

Old and new biomarker research is essential in sepsis to potentially diagnose, monitor, stratify and predict outcome in different diseases, offering the clinician and patient with better prognosis. Therefore, there has been a great deal of interest in developing sepsis-related biomarkers [26].

2.3.3.1. Inflammatory Biomarkers

   a. Procalcitonin. Procalcitonin is currently the most promising diagnostic biomarker for sepsis [26,27]. PCT is a 116-amino-acid peptide and a precursor of calcitonin [27,28]. PCT is normally secreted from the thyroid parafollicular or clear (C) cells, however in sepsis PCT can originate from extra-thyroidal sites including liver, spleen, and adipose tissue [26,28]. Normally, low levels of PCT circulate in the serum -approximately 5-50 pg/ml- but are substantially increased during systemic infections [28,29]. PCT can be detected 2–3 h after an injection of endotoxin in normal human volunteers, and has a half-life of approximately 22-33 h in serum [28,29]. In critically ill patients and pediatric population PCT has consistently demonstrated greater accuracy than C-reactive protein (CRP) in determining sepsis; PCT rises in proportion to the severity of sepsis and reaches its highest levels in septic shock, also tends to be higher in nonsurviror than in survivor [28,30]. PCT demonstrates a wide range of sensitivity and specificity. In a clinical trial, Castelli et al. demonstrated that trauma patients who developed sepsis had higher PCT levels on admission compared with trauma patients who did not develop sepsis, showing a good sensitivity and specifity [31]. However, meta-analysis including a more generalized population of patients in intensive care units, emergency departments (ED), or hospital wards concluded that PCT cannot accurately distinguish sepsis from SIRS [26]. Also studies demonstrate that PCT is useful as a marker in the diagnosis and assessment of severe bacterial infection, but not viral infection [28]. PCT levels were significantly increased in patients with bacterial sepsis compared to controls, but PCT levels were not significantly increased in patients with viral, fungal, or culture negative sepsis compared with controls [26].

b. IL-18. IL-18 is also gaining attention as a potential diagnostic biomarker for sepsis, but the overall data are currently not as robust enough compared to that of PCT [26]. IL-18 is a pro-inflammatory cytokine and a member of the IL-1 super family that activates NF-κB and MAP kinases [32]. Increased IL-18 levels are found in many human inflammatory conditions including rheumatoid arthritis, neonatal infections, and sepsis [26]. Plasma IL-18 levels were significantly increased in patients with sepsis compared to trauma patients on day of admission or at time of sepsis diagnosis. In this same cohort, patients with septic shock had higher IL-18 plasma levels compared to patients without shock. Furthermore, non-survivors with sepsis had significantly higher IL-18 levels compared to survivors from sepsis and IL-18 levels continuously increased during sepsis in non-survivors [26].

c. IL-8. Interleukin-8 is a chemoattractant and activator of neutrophils. Recent evidence suggests that IL-8 can be used to stratify children with septic shock, predicting survival. The initial discovery of IL-8 as a candidate stratification biomarker was in a genome-wide analysis of gene expression using whole blood-derived RNA obtained within 24 hours of admission to the PICU. This microarray-based study revealed that IL-8 was one of the most highly expressed genes in non survivors of pediatric septic shock compared to survivors. Also IL-8 has a negative predictive value for mortality. A serum level of 220 pg/ml, measured within 24 hours of admission to the PICU, may have the ability to predict survival in children with septic shock with 95% probability [26].

d. C reactive protein. CRP has been one of the first biomarkers used to diagnose infection. Its name derived from the fact that it can precipitate from serum in presence of pneumococcal cell wall C-polysaccharide [25]. CRP is an acute-phase reactant released in sepsis and in non-infectious inflammatory disease into the bloodstream from hepatocytes [25,28]. Hepatocyte production is triggered by cytokines, such as IL-1, IL-6 and TNF-α, with striking levels within 4-6 h of the inflammatory stimulus, doubling every 8 h and peaking at around 36-50 h. CRP also has a short half-life of 4-7 h [25]. It is effective, although not perfect, in differentiating between sepsis and non-infectious SIRS [28], and therefore it has also been used to follow response to therapy once an infectious diagnosis has already been established [25]. Owing to its poor specificity, it was often used in combination with other biomarkers as part of a panel of tests to assist clinicians with diagnosis, most notably with PCT and IL-6. Tsalik et al. in a study with ER patients found that PCT, CRP and IL-6 levels were higher in sepsis compared to non-septic patients. Furthermore, biomarker concentrations increased with likelihood of infection and sepsis severity, since ROC curve analysis showed that PCT best predicted septicemia, but CRP better identified clinical infection. Also, a PCT cut off at 0.5 ng/mL had 72.6% sensi- tivity and 69.5% specificity for bacteremia, as well as 40.7% sensitivity and 87.2% specificity for diagnosing infection [33]. In another study, PCT and IL-6 significantly decreased from days 1 to 14 in survivor patients, whereas CRP did not. In non-survivors, the inflammation markers mostly increased within the second week. Also, a logistic regression analysis revealed PCT-POB as an independent determinant for survival. In addition, PCT-POB ≤ 50% (Positive predictive value 75%, sensitivity 97%) and PCT-POB ≤ 25% with CRP-POB ≤ 75% indicated a favorable outcome (Positive predictive value 92% and sensitivity of 67%). Thus, PCT-POB in combination with CRP-POB may serve to monitor efficacy and guide duration of therapy in critically ill patients [34].

e. Natural Killer cells (NK cells). The role of NK cells in sepsis is controversial. NK-cell depletion increases survival and decreases systemic levels of cytokines in experimental models of sepsis. In humans, available data derived from patients in the ICU are scarce, and some of them diverge with the results derived from animal models. Therefore, Andaluz-Ojeda et al. monitored the evolution of NK cells in the blood of patients with severe sepsis and septic shock, demonstrating that compared to survivor patients, non-survivor septic patients showed higher levels of NK cells, in the first 24 hours following admission to the ICU. This suggest that NK cell counts at day 1 are associated with increased risk of mortality in patients who present to the ICU with severe sepsis, abrogating for the prognostic role of NK cells in severe sepsis [35].

2.3.3.2. Oxidative Stress Biomarkers

Critically ill patients suffering from different conditions that may elicit SIRS are at high risk of developing oxidative and nitrosative tissue damage due to a pro-oxidant environment and reduced antioxidant content. These critical conditions cause acute endothelial and mitochondrial dysfunction, thus favouring inflammation, granulocytes activation, increased endothelial permeability, coagulation cascade activation and tissue ischaemia, all of which may further increase reactive oxygen and nitrogen species (RONS) through ischaemia-reperfusion injury cycles [36].

Furthermore, worsening oxidative stress is related to antioxidant vitamin intake below 66% of recommended dietary allowance, thus leading to reduced endogenous levels of substances with antioxidant capacity and further promoting a redox imbalance in critical ill patients [37]. A figure showing the major mechanisms by which RONS are generated under physiologic an pathologic conditions is presented in Figure 1.

In sepsis, increased reactive oxygen species (ROS) may contribute to inflammatory tissue injury through interacting with circulating immune and endothelial cells causing microcirculatory dysfunction. However, recently impaired mitochondrial cellular oxygen utilization, rather than inadequate oxygen delivery, has been claimed to play a more important role in MODS' development [38].

Thus, it seems plausible that ROS could mediate certain pathophysiologic processes during sepsis [39].

Altogether, RONS and biomarkers of either oxidative damage or antioxidant potential could be of use in clinical setting to recognize, evaluate, monitor, mediate and/or predict organ dysfunction development [38].

a. Oxidative damage biomarkers. Since RONS have no specific target and a short half-life, to assess oxidative stress certain oxidation products, as well as micronutrient levels can be measured. The most commonly used biomarkers of oxidative damage are lipid-peroxidation end-products such as: Malondialdehyde (MDA) and F2-isoprostanes [36]. Ware et al. determined that elevated levels of plasma F2-isoprostane and isofuran patients with severe sepsis were associated with renal, hepatic, and coagulation failure; but not with circulatory or pulmonary failure, thus suggesting that they could be useful in monitoring antioxidant treatments [40]. Also, other indicators of oxidative stress have been measured. The thiobarbituric acid reactant substances (TBARS) have been found to be elevated in patients with SIRS and organ dysfunction, and to have a significant correlation with the Sequential Organ Failure Assessment score (SOFA) [41,42]. In addition, Xanthine oxidase activity (XO) has been found to be higher in non-survivor patients. Thus, a level higher than 4 U/mg protein in association with and APACHE II score higher than 20, raised the mortality prediction specificity from 50% to 100% [43]. Similarly, myeloperoxidase activity (MPO) -an enzyme released by activated neutrophils- has been found that is significantly higher in sepsis compared to healthy controls, in conjunction with elevated levels of lactate, TNF-α, IL-8 and IL-1β. All considered, plasma MPO concentrations may constitute a marker of neutrophil proliferation and severity of inflammation [44].

Finally, evidence of elevated nitrosative stress has been found in sepsis. In a rat model of endotoxin-induced inflammation, major NO-derivatives were measured. It was found that nitrite, S- and N-nitrosation and heme-nitrosylation products peaked at 8 h, while nitrate peaked at 12 h. In addition, all of these posttranslational protein modifications were associated with myocardial impairment assessed by echocardiography [45]. Therefore, we can conclude that nitrosative stress may also play a significant role in sepsis pathophysiology, but further investigation is still needed to elucidate the mechanisms by which NO-derivatives may contribute to the clinical features of the disease.

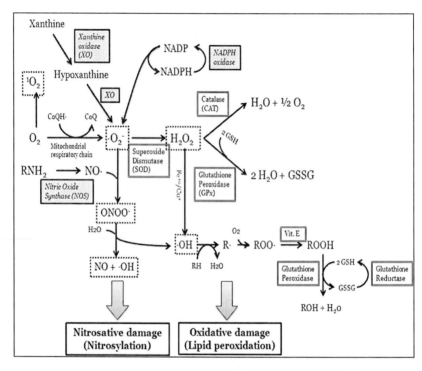

Figure 1. Schematic representation of major reactive oxygen and nitrogen species (RONS) sources and the antioxidant defense system. Superoxide anion (O_2^-) may derive from oxidized oxygen molecules in the mitochondria, from Xanthine metabolism in ATP depletion conditions, from NADPH oxidase activity in activated neutrophils or from lipid peroxidation products. Superoxide dismutase (SOD) metabolize Superoxide anion into hydrogen peroxide (H_2O_2), which in presence of Fe^{+2} or Cu^+ through the Fenton reaction generates hydroxyl radical (OH·), a highy reactive free radical. Hydroxyl radical may damage important biomolecules, especially membrane lipids generating lipid peroxidation products (ROOH). In addition, superoxide anion may react with nitric oxide to form peroxynitrite anion ($ONOO^-$), which in presence of water may further promote oxidative damage as well as nitrosative damage through protein nitrosylation. Antioxidant systems may clear RONS through enzymes mechanisms, such as Catalase (CAT) and Glutathione peroxidase (GPx), or non-enzymatic mechanisms, such as Glutathione (GSH) or antioxidant vitamins (α-tocopherol or β-carotene).

b. Antioxidant potential biomarkers. Antioxidants include special enzymes such as superoxide dismutase (SOD), catalase (CAT) and glutathione peroxidase (GPx, including their cofactors Se, Zn, Mn, and Fe); SH group donors (i.e. glutathione, GSH) and their precursors (i.e. glutamine), and vitamins (i.e. vitamins E and C, and β-carotene) [36].

In patients with septic shock, it has been long found that antioxidant vitamin concentrations, such as: retinol, tocopherol, plasma b-carotene and lycopene, are significantly lower compared to a group of healthy controls [42]. Also, in these patients bilirubin and uric acid have been found to be the most relevant antioxidants [46]. Additionally, the plasma antioxidant potential has been found to be decreased in septic patients who develop organ dysfunction. However, the decrease in plasma antioxidant potential in non-survivors compared to survivors was higher. Also a rapid recovery to normal or supranormal values was observed in survivors, as opposed to non-survivors where increases in plasma antioxidant potential remained below those levels [47].

Also, it has been found that plasma carbonyls and SOD activity are significantly increased in non-survivors. Furthermore, SOD activity correlates significantly with APACHE II score, and presented a similar area under the ROC curve to predict mortality [48]. Recently, Forceville et al. found that plasma Selenoprotein-P (Sel-P) concentrations were 70% lower in patients with septic shock or SIRS with organ dysfunction than in non-SIRS patients and healthy volunteers, while GPx remained unchanged [49].

Finally, plasma redox status has been related to severity. Thus, plasma total antioxidant capacity shows a positive relation to higher APACHE II scores [50,51].

CONCLUSION

Despite recent advances in critical care units, sepsis remains as a prevalent pathology within ICU's and is associated with elevated rates of morbidity, mortality and costs. As mencioned by the SSC statement, to increase survival rates and to improve clinical outcomes in sepsis, focus should be centered in early and accurate recognition of risk factors in septic patients that may improve diagnostic rates and thus lead to on-time effective antimicrobial, fluid resuscitation and goal-directed therapies. Additional tests should be directed to evaluate the current clinical status of the patient, establish a clinical baseline for follow-up, and stratify patients into different groups of severity progression and to confirm the causative pathogen and its antimicrobial spectrum of sensitivity. Inflammatory biomarkers, such as: CRP, PCT, IL-6, IL-8 and IL-

18, as well as NK cells, have been shown to be elevated in sepsis, but are inadequate to discriminate independently as diagnostic tools. In this context, emerging biomarkers of oxidative damage and of antioxidant capacity may provide additional information as well as new insights into sepsis' pathophysiology and have been shown to correlate with clinical scores. However, international guidelines and clinical behavior has paid little attention to its impact. Further research is still necessary to clarify the exact pathophysiological mechanisms by which oxidative and nitrosative stress contribute to sepsis progression, the role of oxidative stress biomarkers and the effects of antioxidant potential enhancement strategies on patients.

REFERENCES

[1] Bone R, Balk R, Cerra F, et al. Definitions for sepsis and organ failure and guidelines for the use of innovative therapies in sepsis. The ACCP/SCCM Consensus Conference Committee. American College of Chest Physicians/Society of Critical Care Medicine. *Chest* 1992; 101:1644-1655.

[2] Levy MM, Fink MP, Marshall JC, et al. 2001 SCCM/ESICM/ACCP/ATS/SIS International Sepsis Definitions Conference. *Intensive Care Med.* 2003; 29:530-8.

[3] Lever A, Mackenzie I. Sepsis: definition, epidemiology, and diagnosis. *BMJ* 2007; 335:879-883.

[4] Goldstein B, Giroir B, Randolph A, and members of the ICC on PS. Internacional pediatric sepsis consensus conference□: Definitions for sepsis and organ dysfunction in pediatrics. *Pediatr Crit. Care Med.* 2005; 6:2-8.

[5] Slade E, Tamber PS, Vincent JL. The Surviving Sepsis Campaign: raising awareness to reduce mortality. *Crit. Care* 2003; 7:1-2.

[6] Annane D, Aegerter P, Jars-Guincestre MC, Guidet B. Current epidemiology of septic shock: the CUB-Réa Network. *Am. J. Respir. Crit. Care Med.* 2003; 168:165-72.

[7] Qureshi K, Rajah A. Septic Shock: A Review Article. *BJMP* 2008; 1:7-12.

[8] Esper AM, Martin GS. Extending international sepsis epidemiology: the impact of organ dysfunction. *Crit. Care* 2009; 13:120.

[9] Vincent JL, Sakr Y, Sprung CL, Ranieri VM, Reinhart K, Gerlach H, Moreno R, Carlet J, Le Gall JR PD. Sepsis in European intensive care units: results of the SOAP study. *Crit. Care Med.* 2006; 34:344-353.
[10] Barie PS HL. Epidemiology of multiple organ dysfunction syndrome in critical surgical illness. *Surg Infect* 2000; 1:173-185.
[11] Zhang SW, Wang H, Su Q, Wang BE, Wang C YC. [Clinical epidemiology of 1,087 patients with multiple organ dysfunction syndrome]. *Zhongguo Wei Zhong Bing Ji Jiu Yi Xue.* 2007; 19:2-6.
[12] Silva E, Araujo DV. Economic and Social Burden of Severe Sepsis. In: Vincent J-L, ed. Yearbook of Intensive Care and Emergency Medicine. Springer-Verlag Berlin Heidelberg, 2009: 129-140.
[13] Ward NS, Casserly B, Ayala A. The Compensatory Anti-inflammatory Response syndrome (CARS) in Critically ill patients. *Clin. Chest Med.* 2008; 29:617.
[14] Hotchkiss RS, Karl IE. The pathophysiology and treatment of sepsis. *N. Engl. J. Med.* 2003; 348:138-50.
[15] Wang Z, Schorr C, Hunter K, Dellinger R. Contrasting treatment and outcomes of septic shock: presentation on hospital floors versus emergency department. *Chin. Med. J.* 2010; 123:3550-3553.
[16] Band R a, Gaieski DF, Hylton JH, Shofer FS, Goyal M, Meisel ZF. Arriving by emergency medical services improves time to treatment endpoints for patients with severe sepsis or septic shock. *Acad. Emerg. Med.* 2011; 18:934-40.
[17] Rangel-Frausto MS, Pittet D, Hwang T, Woolson RF, Wenzel RP. The dynamics of disease progression in sepsis: Markov modeling describing the natural history and the likely impact of effective antisepsis agents. *CID* 1998; 27:185-90.
[18] Alberti C, Brun-Buisson C, Chevret S, et al. Systemic inflammatory response and progression to severe sepsis in critically ill infected patients. *Am. J. Respir. Crit. Care Med.* 2005; 171:461-8.
[19] Nguyen HB, Rivers EP, Abrahamian FM, et al. Severe sepsis and septic shock: review of the literature and emergency department management guidelines. *Ann. Emerg. Med.* 2006; 48:28-54.
[20] Talan D a, Moran GJ, Abrahamian FM. Severe sepsis and septic shock in the emergency department. *Infect Dis. Clin. N. Am.* 2008; 22:1-31.
[21] Hajjar LA, Nakamura RE, Almeida JPD, et al. Lactate and base deficit are predictors of mortality in critically ill patients with cancer. *Clinics* 2011; 66:2037-2042.

[22] Wendel M, Heller a R, Koch T. [Pathomechanisms of organ failure. Mitochondrial dysfunction in sepsis]. *Der Anaesthesist* 2009; 58:343-52.
[23] Dellinger RP, Levy MM, Carlet JM, et al. Surviving Sepsis Campaign: international guidelines for management of severe sepsis and septic shock: 2008. *Crit. Care Med.* 2008; 36:296-327.
[24] Tsiotou AG, Sakorafas GH, Anagnostopoulos G, Bramis J. Septic shock; current pathogenetic concepts from a clinical perspective. *Med. Sci. Monit.* 2005; 11:76-85.
[25] Standage SW, Wong HR. Biomarkers for pediatric sepsis and septic shock. *Expert Rev. Anti. Infect Ther.* 2011; 9:71-79.
[26] Kaplan J, Wong H. Biomarker discovery and development in pediatric critical care medicine. *Pediatr Crit. Care Med.* 2011; 12:165-173.
[27] Snider R, Nylen E, Becker K. Procalcitonin and its component peptides in systemic inflammation: immunochemical characterization. *J. Investig. Med.* 1997; 45:552-560.
[28] Mitaka C. Clinical laboratory differentiation of infectious versus non-infectious systemic inflammatory response syndrome. *Clin. Chim. Acta* 2005; 351:17-29.
[29] Assicot M, Gendrel D, Carsin H, Raymond J, Guilbaud J, Bohuon C. High serum procalcitonin concentrations in patients with sepsis and infection. *Lancet* 1993; 341:515-518.
[30] Hoeboer SH, Alberts E, van den Hul I, Tacx AN, Debets-Ossenkopp YJ, Groeneveld a BJ. Old and new biomarkers for predicting high and low risk microbial infection in critically ill patients with new onset fever: A case for procalcitonin. *J. Infect* 2012; 64:484-493.
[31] Castelli G, Pognani C, Cita M, Paladini R. Procalcitonin as a prognostic and diagnostic tool for septic complications after major trauma. *Crit. Care Med.* 2009; 37:1845-1849.
[32] Tschoeke S, Oberholzer A, Moldawer L. Interleukin-18: a novel prognostic cytokine in bacteria-induced sepsis. *Crit. Care Med.* 2006; 34:1225-1233.
[33] Tsalik EL, Jaggers LB, Glickman SW, et al. Discriminative Value of Inflammatory Biomarkers for Suspected Sepsis. *J. Emerg. Med.* 2011;: [Epub ahead of print].
[34] Tschaikowsky K, Hedwig-Geissing M, Braun GG, Radespiel-Troeger M. Predictive value of procalcitonin, interleukin-6, and C-reactive protein for survival in postoperative patients with severe sepsis. *J. Crit. Care.* 2011; 26:54-64.

[35] Andaluz-Ojeda D, Iglesias V, Bobillo F, et al. Early natural killer cell counts in blood predict mortality in severe sepsis. *Crit. Care* 2011; 15:R243.
[36] Bernal ME, Varon J, Acosta P, Montagnier L. Oxidative stress in critical care medicine. *Int. J. Clin. Pract.* 2010; 64:1480-1488.
[37] Abilés J, de la Cruz AP, Castaño J, et al. Oxidative stress is increased in critically ill patients according to antioxidant vitamins intake, independent of severity: a cohort study. *Crit. Care* 2006; 10:R146.
[38] Saa D, Rodrigo R. Pathophysiology of Multiple Organ Dysfunction Syndrome in sepsis. In: Rodrigo R, von Dessauer B, eds. Oxidative stress and the critically ill patient. Nova Science Publishers, 2012: in press.
[39] von Dessauer B, Bongain J, Molina V, Quilodrán J, Castillo R, Rodrigo R. Oxidative stress as a novel target in pediatric sepsis management. *J. Crit. Care.* 2011; 26:103.e1-7.
[40] Ware L, Fessel J, May A, Roberts L. Plasma biomarkers of oxidant stress and development of organ failure in severe sepsis. *Shock* 2011; 36:12-17.
[41] Motoyama T, Okamoto K, Kukita I, Hamaguchi M, Kinoshita Y, Ogawa H. Possible role of increased oxidant stress in multiple organ failure after systemic inflammatory response syndrome. *Crit. Care Med.* 2003; 31:1048-1052.
[42] Goode H, Cowley H, Walker B, Howdle P, Webster N. Decreased antioxidant status and increased lipid peroxidation in patients with septic shock and secondary organ dysfunction. *Crit. Care Med.* 1995; 23:646-651.
[43] Luchtemberg MN, Petronilho F, Constantino L, et al. Xanthine oxidase activity in patients with sepsis. *Clinical biochemistry* 2008; 41:1186-90.
[44] Kothari N, Keshari RS, Bogra J, et al. Increased myeloperoxidase enzyme activity in plasma is an indicator of inflammation and onset of sepsis. *J. Crit. Care.* 2011; 26:435.e1-435.e7.
[45] Dyson A, Bryan NS, Fernandez BO, et al. An integrated approach to assessing nitroso-redox balance in systemic inflammation. *Free Radic. Biol. Med.* 2011; 51:1137-45.
[46] Pascual C, Karzai W, Meier-Hellmann A, et al. Total plasma antioxidant capacity is not always decreased in sepsis. *Crit. Care Med.* 1998; 26:705-709.

[47] Cowley H, Bacon P, Goode H, Webster N, Jones J, Menon D. Plasma antioxidant potential in severe sepsis: a comparison of survivors and nonsurvivors. *Crit. Care Med.* 1996; 24:1179-1183.

[48] Guerreiro M, Petronilho F, Andrades M, et al. Plasma superoxide dismutase activity and mortality in septic patients [corrected]. *J. Trauma.* 2010; 69:E102-106.

[49] Forceville X, Mostert V, Pierantoni A, et al. Selenoprotein P, rather than glutathione peroxidase, as a potential marker of septic shock and related syndromes. *Eur Surg Res* 2009; 43:338-47.

[50] Alonso de Vega J, Díaz J, Serrano E, Carbonell L. Plasma redox status relates to severity in critically ill patients. *Crit. Care Med.* 2000; 28:1812-1814.

[51] Chuang C-C, Shiesh S-C, Chi C-H, et al. Serum total antioxidant capacity reflects severity of illness in patients with severe sepsis. *Crit. Care* 2006; 10:R36.

In: Septic Shock
Editors: M. Johnston and J. Knight

ISBN: 978-1-62257-485-8
© 2012 Nova Science Publishers, Inc.

Chapter 4

DIAGNOSIS AND MANAGEMENT OF LIFE-THREATENING INFECTIONS AND SEPTIC SHOCK DURING IDIOPATHIC DRUG-INDUCED AGRANULOCYTOSIS

Emmanuel Andrès[1*]*, Jacques Zimmer*[2]*, Khalid Serraj*[3] *and Frédéric Maloisel*[4]

[1]Departments of Internal Medicine B, University Hospital of Strasbourg, Strasbourg, France
[2]Laboratory of Immunogenetics and Allergology, Centre de Recherche Public de la Santé (CRP-Santé), Luxembourg-City Luxembourg
[3]Department of Internal Medicine and Hematology, University Hospital of Oujda, Oujda, Maroc
[4]Department of Hematology, Saint Anne's Clinic, Strasbourg, France

---

[*] Pr E. ANDRÈS, Service de Médecine Interne, Clinique Médicale B, Hôpital Civil, *Hôpitaux Universitaires de Strasbourg*, 1 Porte de l'Hôpital, 67 091 Strasbourg Cedex, FRANCE. Phone: 33-3-88-11-50-66. Fax: 33-3-88-11-62-62. Mail: emmanuel.andres@chru-strasbourg.fr

Abstract

In this chapter, we report and discuss the diagnosis and management of life-threatening infections and septic shock during acute and severe neutropenia (neutrophil count of <0.5 x 10^9/L) related to drug intake. This rare event, called "idiopathic agranulocytosis", remains a potentially serious adverse event of drugs due to the presence of severe deep tissue infections (e.g., pneumonia), septicemia, and septic shock in approximately two-thirds of the patients. Recently, several prognostic factors have been identified that may be helpful when identifying "frailty" patients. Old age (>65 years), septicemia or shock, metabolic disorders such as renal failure, and a neutrophil count below 0.1×10^9/L have been consensually accepted as poor prognostic factors. In this potentially life-threatening disorder, modern management with broad-spectrum antibiotics and hematopoietic growth factors (particularly *G-CSF*), is likely to improve the prognosis. Thus, with appropriate management, the mortality rate of idiosyncratic drug-induced agranulocytosis is currently around 5%.

Keywords: Agranulocytosis. Neutropenia. Idiosyncratic drug-induced agranulocytosis. Infections. Antibiotics. Hematopoietic growth factor

Introduction

Agranulocytosis or acute neutropenia are characterized by a profound decrease or an absolute lack of circulating granulocytes, classically resulting in a neutrophil count of <0.5 x 10^9/L [1,2]. The term 'agranulocytosis' was first introduced in 1922 by Schultz for cases of acute and severe pharyngeal infections, associated with a lack of granulocytes in the blood. In the majority of patients, the neutrophil count is under 0.1 x 10^9/L.

Patients with such severe acute neutropenia are at high risk of developing complications such as pyrexia, but also of severe or life-threatening and sometimes fatal infections [2, 3].

In this chapter, we report and discuss the diagnosis and management of life-threatening infections and septic shock during acute and severe neutropenia.

Criteria for the Definition of Idiopathic Drug-Induced Agranulocytosis

Most, but not all cases of agranulocytosis occur as a result of exposure to drugs: chemotherapy (chemotherapy induced-agranulocytosis), immune modulator agents or biotherapies, or other drugs; the latter case represents "idiosyncratic drug-induced agranulocytosis", as we have previously published in *Expert Opinion in Hematology* [4]. Either the drug itself or one of its metabolites may be the causative agent [5].

Currently, the recommended criteria for diagnosing blood cytopenias and for implicating a drug as a causative agent in neutropenia are derived from an international consensus meeting [2,6]. These criteria are outlined in *table 1*.

Table 1. Criteria for idiosyncratic drug-induced agranulocytosis [2,3,6]

Definition of agranulocytosis:	Criteria of drug imputability:
	• Onset of agranulocytosis during treatment or within 7 days of exposure to the drug, with a complete recovery in neutrophil count of more than 1.5×10^9/L within one month of discontinuing the drug
	• Recurrence of agranulocytosis upon re-exposure to the drug (this is rarely observed, as the high risk of mortality contra-indicates redamministration of the drug)
	• Exclusion criteria: history of congenital neutropenia or immune mediated neutropenia, recent infectious disease (particularly recent viral infection), recent chemotherapy and/or radiotherapy and/or immunotherapy* and existence of an underlying hematological disease

*Immunoglobulins, interferon, anti-TNF antibodies, anti-CD20 (rituximab).

Epidemiology of Agranulocytosis

Idiosyncratic drug-induced agranulocytosis is a rare disorder. In Europe, the annual incidence of such events is between 1.6 and 9.2 cases per million population [3,7-10]. In the USA, reported rates rang from 2.4 to 15.4 per million per year [11].

In our experience (observational study in a French hospital), from 1996 to 2003, the annual incidence of symptomatic idiosyncratic drug-induced agranulocytosis remained stable, with approximately 6 cases per million population [12].

Differences in the incidence may be due to different methods/inclusion criteria used in the studies published [3,6].

It's important to keep in mind that the incidence remains unchanged, despite the withdrawn of incriminated drugs (which carry a high risk of idiosyncratic drug induced neutropenia) and increased levels of medical awareness and pharmacovigilence [6].

INCRIMINATED DRUGS IN IDIOPATHIC AGRANULOCYTOSIS

Firstly, it is important to note that almost all classes of drugs have been implicated [2,3,12-16], but for the majority the risk appears to be very small [3].

However, for drugs such as antithyroid medications, ticlopidine, clozapine, sulfasalazine, trimethoprim-sulfametoxazole (cotrimoxazole) and dipyrone, the risk may be higher [3,17,18]. For example, for antithyroid drugs, a risk of 3 per 10,000 users has been reported [2]. For ticlopidine, the risk is more than 100-fold higher [9]. Clozapine induces agranulocytosis in almost 1% of patients, particularly in the first three months of treatment, with older patients and females being at a higher risk [18].

In our single center cohort previously published in *The European Journal of Internal Medicine*, the most frequent causative drugs were [12]:

- antibiotics (25%), particularly β-lactams and cotrimoxazole, which has strong implications on the management of this event (cross-reactivity of antibiotic molecules);
- antithyroid drugs such as neomercazole (23%);

- antiplatelet agents such as ticlopidine (16%);
- neuroleptic and antiepileptic agents (11%);
- and nonsteroidal anti-inflammatory agents (8%).

These findings are similar to two recent reports that incriminated the same drug families [17,19]. These drug families are outlined in *figure 1*.

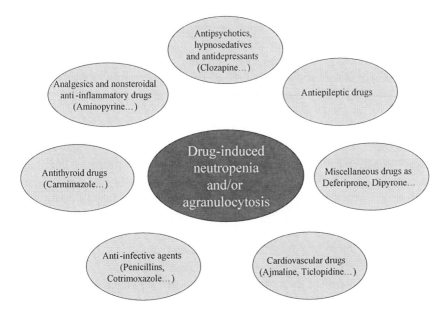

Figure 1. Drugs implicated in the occurrence of agranulocytosis [2,3].

In our cohort study, two thirds of patients received more than two drugs with a mean of three drugs, accounting for the difficulty in definitively identifying the drug responsible fir the agranulocytosis. In this cohort, no over (the-counter medications (*"self medication"*) were implicated [11]. No inappropriate prescribing, as the use of drug that pose more risk than benefit, the misuse of drugs by dose or duration, is also identified.

Clinical Manifestations of Drug-Induced Neutropenia and Agranulocytosis

Initially, patients with drug-induced acute neutropenia or agranulocytosis usually present with fever, which often is the earliest and sometimes the only sign during evolution, associated with general malaise, often including chills [2, 3, 14, 20]. They also commonly present a non-specific sore throat. More rarely, patients have first, as a not expected and brutal event, a severe deep and potentially life-threatening infection (as *"un coup de tonnerre dans un ciel serein"*) [3]. It's important to note that without medical intervention, particularly immediate antibiotics administration, most patients (>60% in our experience) develop severe and potentially life-threatening infections with signs of general sepsis and septicemia (fever, chills, hypotension...), while some have clinical signs of pneumonia as well as anorectal, skin or oropharyngeal infections and septic shock [2, 3, 13, 14, 20]. Clinicians must keep in mind that the signs of these infections are often crude and atypical because of the neutropenia (e.g. no purulent sputum, no image on X-ray for pneumonia...) [2]. In patients receiving chemotherapy for the treatment of cancer, the occurrence and type of infections (bacterial or fungal) depends on the degree and duration of the neutropenia [2, 21]. It is notable that when antibiotics are administered prophylactically, or at the beginning of this adverse event, both the patient's complaints and the physical findings may be "masked" and fever is often the only clinical sign detected [2, 11]. The clinical presentations recorded in our cohort study of hospitalized patients with idiosyncratic drug-induced agranulocytosis included [12]:

- isolated fever (41%);
- septicemia and septic shock (34%);
- pneumonia (10%);
- sore throat and acute tonsillitis (7%);
- cutaneous infections (4%);
- other deep tissue infections (4%).

Thus, in this cohort, clinical manifestations included septicemia or septic shock and other severe infections in one-third and one-quarter of patients respectively.

A causative pathogen, typically Gram-negative bacilli or Gram-positive cocci (mainly *Staphylococcus spp.*), was isolated in 30% of cases in one series [2]. Fungi are also involved as secondary infective agents (>10%).

It is worth noting, that in elderly patients, clinical manifestations were generally more severe, with septicemia or septic shock in at least two-thirds of patients in our experience, as we have previously published in *The American Journal of Medicine* and in *Drugs Aging* [22,23].

At the opposite side, some patients (<20%), with not-well identified characteristics or profile, remained asymptomatic [2,3,24]. This supports the case for routine monitoring of blood counts in individuals receiving high-risk medications such as antithyroid drugs, as recommended by Tajiri *et al* [24,25], or ticlopidine [3,]. This also supports a not consensual home management of such an event in certain patients (young, without medical history, with fever as the sole sign) [2,3].

Differential Diagnosis of Acute Neutropenia

The differential diagnosis of acute neutropenia in adults includes a limited number of conditions [2].

In practice and in the literature, acute neutropenia disorder has been shown to be attributable to drugs in 70 to 90% of cases [2-4]. In the Berlin prospective Case-Control Surveillance Study of Serious Rare Blood Dyscrasias, acute agranulocytosis was found to be drug-related in 97% of cases as reported by Andersohn *et al* [4].

Thus in practice, drug-induced neutropenia or agranulocytosis should be discussed routinely (considered in first) even if there is a context moving towards another condition.

In this context, *the* clinician must keep in mind that in all cases, the patient's medication history must be carefully obtained in chronological order so that the suspected agent(s) may be identified [2]. Theoretically, acute neutropenia is classically diagnosed in a blood sample, resulting in a neutrophil count of <0.5 x 10^9/L, [1,2].

In the majority of patients, the neutrophil count is under 0.1 x 10^9/L. Nevertheless, in our experience, bone marrow examination may be required in all patients to exclude an underlying pathology, especially in the elderly [25]. In such patients, the bone marrow typically shows a lack of mature myeloid cells, whereas in other cases, immature cells from the myelocyte stage are preserved.

This latter appearance is described as "myeloid maturation arrest" [2]. In clinical practice, the main differential diagnoses include in adults:

- neutropenia secondary to sepsis, particularly viral infections or bacterial infections (severe Gram negative infections with *Salmonella sp.*, tuberculosis, *Brucella sp.*);
- neutropenia manifesting as the first sign of bone marrow failure - such as in myelodysplastic syndromes;
- neutropenia associated with hypersplenism [2, 12].
- Other, rarer differential diagnoses include neutropenia secondary to nutritional deficiencies, Felty's syndrome, systemic lupus erythematosus or Sjögren's syndrome [2, 12].

PROGNOSIS AND MORTALITY RATE OF DRUG INDUCED AGRANULOCYTOSIS, FRAILTY PATIENTS

Over the past twenty years, the mortality rate for idiosyncratic drug-induced agranulocytosis or severe neutropenia was 10-16% in European studies [2, 13, 21].

However, this has recently fallen to 5% (range, 2.5 to 10%). This is likely due to improved recognition, management and treatment of the condition as demonstrated by Andersohn *et al* and our team [2, 3, 12]. The highest mortality rate is observed in frailty patients: older patients (>65 years), as well as those with renal failure (defined as serum creatinine level >120 µmol/L), bacteraemia or shock at diagnosis or low neutrophil count levels, as firstly reported by Julia *et al* [2, 21, 26].

We have recently confirmed these findings by performing a uni- and multivariate analysis of factors affecting the outcome in our cohort study (n = 91) [26].

In particular, we found that a neutrophil count of <0.1 x 10^9/L at diagnosis, as well as septicemia and/or shock, were variables that were significantly associated with a longer neutrophil recovery time.

In our cohort, bone marrow showing a lack of myeloid cells was not found to be associated with a delayed recovery (using uni- and multivariate analysis) [26]. In contrast, the use of hematopoietic growth factors was associated with a shorter neutrophil recovery time (*see the next section*).

In a recent systematic review by Andersohn *et al* [3], which included 492 published case reports of agranulocytosis, it was shown that patients with a neutrophil count of <0.1 x 10^9/L had a higher rate of localized infections (59% versus 39%, *p* <0.001), sepsis (20% versus 6%, *p* <0.001) and fatal complications (10% versus 3%, *p* <0.001) than those with a neutrophil nadir ≥0.1 x 10^9/L.

Management of Drug-Induced Severe Neutropenia or Agranulocytosis

Prevention
In our opinion, routine monitoring in patients taking medications with a confirmed, albeit rare association with neutropenia or agranulocytosis, is not worthwhile [2]. However, routine monitoring for agranulocytosis *is* required in some high-risk drugs, such as clozapine, ticlopidine and antithyroid drugs [2,6,24,25].

General Measures
The management of idiosyncratic drug-induced neutropenia begins with the immediate withdrawal of any medications, which may potentially be responsible [2,12,13]. The patient's medication history must be carefully obtained in chronological order so that the suspected agent(s) may be identified.

Importantly, the appropriate pharmacovigilence center must be notified of all cases of drug-induced neutropenia or agranulocytosis [3].

Patients at high risk of infection (frailty patients, with regard to the prognosis of drug-induced neutropenia [*see the section below*]) should be admitted to hospital, without any delay (*figure 2*) [3,27].

It should be noted that as a result of neutrophil deficiency, both the patient's symptoms and the physical findings may be altered, and fever may be the only clinical sign (*see the section clinical manifestations*) [26].

Important prognostic factors resulting in an increased risk of serious complications must be systematically searched [22].

Patients with a low risk of infection, with none of the bad factors of prognosis and good performance status, should also usually be treated in hospital, unless adequate and comprehensive medical follow-up can be provided in an ambulatory setting or at home (*figure 2*) [2,3,27]. Nevertheless to date, several not frailty patients are managed in home with intensive supervision and monitoring!

Concomitant measures include aggressive treatment of confirmed or potential sepsis, as well as the prevention of secondary infections [2,20].

Preventive measures include good hygiene and infection control, paying particular attention to high-risk areas such as the mouth, skin and perineum [2,12]. Patient isolation and the use of prophylactic antibiotics (e.g. for the gastrointestinal tract) have been proposed, but their usefulness in limiting the risk of infection has not been documented or at least, has not been clinically proven [2].

In case of fever or signs of sepsis, multiple bacterial samples should be collected, systematically and in all suspected sites of infection, as blood, urine and stool cultures [2,3,27]. After one week of fever, deep and invasive mycosis (candidosis, aspergillosis, mucormycosis) should also be screened systematically with appropriate microbial technologies.

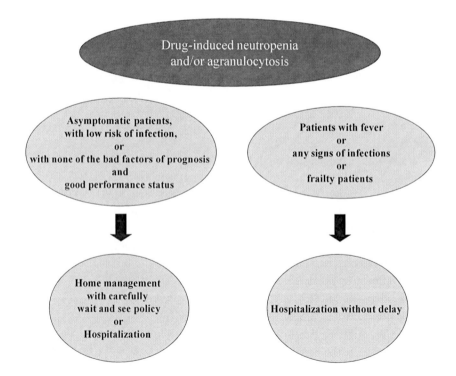

Figure 2. Management of patients with drug-induced neutropenia and agranulocytosis [2,3,27].

Indications of Antimicrobial Agents

In our experience, severe infections were diagnosed in more than 60% of the patients and Gram-negative bacilli or Gram-positive cocci (mainly *Staphylococcus spp.*) were isolated in 30% of cases and fungi in around 10% [2,12]. Thus, the occurrence of sepsis in drug-induced agranulocytosis requires prompt management, without any delay, including the administration of broad-spectrum intravenous antibiotic therapy (after blood, urine and any other relevant samples have been drawn for culture [2,12,13,20]).

Empiric, broad-spectrum antibacterial therapy is generally the best choice, but the choice of antibiotic used may need to be adapted depending on the nature of the sepsis, the clinical status of the patient, local patterns of antibiotic resistance and previous antibiotic use [2,20].

In our hospital, we commonly combine in first line therapy, new cephalosporins and quinolones or aminoglycosides [12,22]. Of course ureidopenicillins beta-lactam/beta-lactamase inhibitor combinations, as carbapenems, or imipenem can be safely used in these antibiotic combinations [2,3,27].

The addition of intravenous vancomycin or teicoplanin is considered in patients at high risk of serious gram-positive infections or after 48 hours of continued fever despite first line of antibiotics with at least cephalosporins [2,3,27]. When an antibiotic is suspected of being the causative agent resulting in neutropenia, one should keep in mind the potential for antibody cross-reactivity, and therefore the choice of further antibiotics to be administered should be considered very carefully [2,3]. In patients with a persistent fever despite broad-spectrum antibiotics against Gram-negative bacilli or Gram-positive cocci or systematically after 1 week of persistent fever, the addition of empirical antifungal agents should be considered, as amphotericin B or related derivates (e.g. liposomal preparation of amphotericin) and voriconazol or caspofungin [20,27].

It's important to note that these recommendations are not validated specifically for idiosyncratic drug-induced neutropenia or agranulocytosis but are based on the evidence based-medicine recommendations for the management of chemotherapy-induced neutropenia (field of oncology) [2,3].

It's also important to keep in mind that transfusions of granulocyte concentrates should only be used in exceptional circumstances, and only then for the control of life-threatening infections with antibiotic resistance - such as perineal gangrene [2].

Indications of Hematopoietic *Growth Factors*

In idiosyncratic drug-induced severe neutropenia or agranulocytosis, the use of hematopoietic growth factors such as *Granulocyte-* and *Granulocyte-Macrophage-Colony Stimulating factor* (*G-CSF and GM-CSF*) has been previously reported [22,28-31]. Since 1985, two-thirds of reported cases of drug-induced agranulocytosis have been treated with hematopoietic growth factors [3,32]. The most recent, major studies on hematopoietic growth factor use in drug-induced agranulocytosis are described in table 2 [3,22,29-32].

It is of note that most of the data regarding the efficacy of these hematopoietic growth factors comes from case reports and case series using a comparison control group obtained from historic data [2,3,20].

Nevertheless, in our opinion, it may be to date unethical to study the effects of these growth factors using the criteria for evidence-based medicine i.e. prospective controlled randomized trials. In fact in our experience, *G-CSF* and *GM-CSF* (at a mean dose of 300 µg/day) were found to be useful in shortening the duration of blood count recovery time, without inducing any major toxic or adverse effects, particularly in patients with poor prognostic factors (frailty patients described below) [22,26,28,33].

Moreover in a multivariate analysis of all our cases of idiosyncratic drug-induced agranulocytosis (published in *Haematologica*), we demonstrated that hematopoietic growth factor (*G-CSF*) use was an independent variable, which positively affected the duration of hematological recovery time [22].

We also demonstrated that the duration of antibiotic therapy and hospital stay were significantly shorter in patients treated with hematopoietic growth factors [22,28].

In this cohort study, we also established the long-term (mean follow-up >52 months) safety of hematopoietic growth factors, in the absence of hematological adverse events such as myelodysplasia and hematological proliferative disorders [34].

The recent systematic review of all published case reports of non-chemotherapy drug-induced agranulocytosis by Andersohn *et al* [3] published in *The Annals of Internal Medicine* confirms this data. A recent study by Ibanez *et al* (Barcelona cohort) also concludes that *G-CSF* shortens recovery time in patients with agranulocytosis [31]. However, it's important to note that only one study reported a lower mortality rate with this therapy [30].

Table 2. Recent Studies on the Use of Hematopoietic Growth Factors In Idiosyncratic Drug-Induced Agranulocytosis (*Adapted From* [2, 6, 20])

Type of study and target population	Main results
Systematic review of all published cases (n = 492); All patients with idiosyncratic drug-induced agranulocytosis [3]	Treatment with hematopoietic growth factors was associated with a statistically significantly lower rate of infectious and fatal complications, in cases with a neutrophil count <0.1 x 10^9/L
Meta-analysis (n = 118); All patients with idiosyncratic drug-induced agranulocytosis [30]	G-CSF or GM-CSF (100 to 600 μg/day) reduced the mean time to neutrophil recovery (neutrophil count >0.5 x 10^9/L) from 10 to 7.7 days, in cases with a neutrophil count <0.1 x 10^9/L, and reduced the mortality rate from 16 to 4.2%
Case control study, retrospective analysis (n = 70); All patients with idiosyncratic drug-induced agranulocytosis [29]	G-CSF and GM-CSF (100 to 600 μg/day) reduced the recovery of neutrophil count from 7 to 4 days, particularly in patients with a neutrophil count <0.1 x 10^9/L
Cohort study, retrospective analysis (n = 54); Patients with idiosyncratic drug-induced agranulocytosis >65 years of age, with poor prognostic factors [22]	G-CSF (300 μg/day) significantly reduced the mean duration for hematological recovery from 8.8 to 6.6 days (p <0.04). G-CSF reduced the global cost
Cohort study, retrospective analysis (n = 20); Patients with antithyroid drug-induced agranulocytosis and poor prognostic factors [28]	G-CSF (300 μg/day) significantly reduced the mean durations of hematological recovery, antibiotic therapy and hospitalization from: 11.6 to 6.8 days, 12 to 7.5 days and 13 to 7.3 days, respectively (p <0.05 in all cases). G-CSF reduced the global cost
Cohort study, retrospective analysis (n = 145); All patients with idiosyncratic drug-induced agranulocytosis [31]	G-CSF shortens time to recovery in patients with agranulocytosis
Prospective randomized study (n = 24); All patients with antithyroid drug-induced agranulocytosis [32]	G-CSF (100 to 200 μg/day) did not significantly reduce the mean duration for hematological recovery

G-CSF: Granulocyte-Colony Stimulating factor. GM-CSF: Granulocyte-Macrophage-Colony Stimulating factor.

It's important to keep in mind in an evidence based medicine perspective that the only prospective randomized study available did not confirm the benefit of *G-CSF* [32]. A total of 24 patients with antithyroid-related drug-induced agranulocytosis were enrolled, it is likely that both the small size of the study and the administration of an inappropriately low dose of *G-CSF* (100 to 200 µg/day) contributed to these negative results.

CONCLUSION

To date, idiosyncratic drug-induced agranulocytosis or acute severe neutropenia remains a potentially serious adverse event due to the frequency of severe sepsis with severe deep tissue infections (e.g., pneumonia), life threatening infections, septicemia, and septic shock in two-thirds of all hospitalized patients. However, several prognostic factors have recently been identified which may be helpful when identifying "susceptible" or frailty patients. Old age (>65 years), septicemia or shock, metabolic disorders such as renal failure and a neutrophil count below 0.1×10^9/L have been consensually accepted as poor prognostic factors.

In this potentially life-threatening disorder, modern management with broad-spectrum antibiotics and hematopoietic growth factors as *G-CSF*, is likely to improve the prognosis. Thus with appropriate management, the mortality rate from idiosyncratic drug-induced agranulocytosis is currently around 5%.

No sources of funding were used to assist the preparation of this manuscript. The authors have no conflicts of interest that are directly relevant of the content of this manuscript. E. Andrès is recipient of a grant from *CHUGAI, AMGEN, ROCHE, GSK, BMS, GENZYME,* ACTELION, *VIFOR* but these sponsors had no part in the research or writing of the present manuscript. E. Andrès is a member of the French national commission of pharmacovigilance, but the present manuscript represents individual opinion. F. Maloisel is recipient of a grant from *CHUGAI, AMGEN, ROCHE, SHIRE, GSK* but these sponsors had no part in the research or writing of the present manuscript.

REFERENCES

[1] Bénichou C. Adverse drug reactions. A practical guide to diagnosis and management. New York: WJ Wiley; 1994.
[2] Andrès E, Dali-Youcef N, Serraj K, Zimmer J. Recognition and management of drug-induced blood-cytopenias: the example of idiosyncratic drug-induced thrombocytopenia. *Expert Opin. Drug Saf.* 2009; 8: 183–190.
[3] Andersohn F, Konzen C, Garbe E. Non-chemotherapy drug-induced agranulocytosis: A systematic review of case reports. *Ann. Intern. Med.* 2007; 146: 657-65.
[4] Andrès E, Zimmer J, Mecili M, Weitten T, Alt M. Clinical presentation and management of drug-induced agranulocytosis. *Expert Rev. Hematol.* 2011; 4: 143-151.
[5] Andersohn F, Bronder E, Klimpel A, Garbe E. Proportion of drug-related serious rare blood dyscrasias: estimates from the Berlin Case-Control Surveillance Study. *Am. J. Hematol.* 2004; 77: 316-8.
[6] Bénichou C, Solal-Celigny P. Standardization of definitions and criteria for causality assessment of adverse drug reactions. Drug-induced blood cytopenias: report of an international consensus meeting. *Nouv. Rev. Fr. Hematol.* 1993; 33: 257-62.
[7] Van der Klauw MM, Goudsmit R, Halie MR, van't Veer MB, Herings RM, Wilson JH et al. A population-based case-cohort study of drug-associated agranulocytosis. *Arch Intern Med* 1999; 159: 369-74.
[8] Van Staa TP, Boulton F, Cooper C, Hagenbeek A, Inskip H, Leufkens HG. Neutropenia and agranulocytosis in England and Wales: incidence and risk factors. *Am. J. Hematol.* 2003; 72: 248-54.
[9] Theophile H, Begaud B, Martin K, Laporte JR, Capella D. Incidence of agranulocytosis in Southwest France. *Eur J Epidemiol* 2004; 19: 563-5.
[10] Ibanez L, Vidal X, Ballarin E, Laporte JR. Population-based drug-induced agranulocytosis. *Arch. Intern. Med.* 2005; 165: 869-74.
[11] Strom BL, Carson JL, Schinnar R, Snyder ES, Shaw M. Descriptive epidemiology of agranulocytosis. *Arch. Intern. Med.* 1992; 152: 1475-80.
[12] Andrès E, Maloisel F, Kurtz JE, Kaltenbach G, Alt M, Weber JC et al. Modern management of non-chemotherapy drug-induced agranulocytosis: a monocentric cohort study of 90 cases and review of the literature. *Eur. J. Intern. Med.* 2002; 13: 324-8.

[13] Patton WN, Duffull SB. Idiosyncratic drug-induced haematological abnormalities: incidence, pathogenosis, management and avoidance. *Drug Safety* 1994; 11: 445-62.
[14] Paitel JF, Stockemer V, Dorvaux V, Witz F, Guerci A, Lederlin P. Agranulocytoses aiguës médicamenteuses. Etude clinique à propos de 30 patients et évolution des étiologies sur 2 décennies. *Rev. Med. Interne.* 1995; 16: 495-9.
[15] Vial T, Pofilet C, Pham E, Payen C, Evreux JC. Agranulocytoses aiguës médicamenteuses: expérience du Centre Régional de Pharmacovigilance de Lyon sur 7 ans. *Therapie* 1996; 51: 508-15.
[16] Shapiro S, Issaragrisil S, Kaufman DW, Anderson T, Chansung K, Thamprasit T et al. Agranulocytosis in Bangkok, Thailand: a predominantly drug-induced disease with an unusually low incidence. Aplastic Anemia Study Group. *Am. J. Trop. Med. Hyg.* 1999; 60: 573-7.
[17] Van der Klauw MM, Wilson JH, Stricker BH. Drug-associated agranulocytosis: 20 years of reporting in the Netherlands (1974-1994). *Am. J. Hematol.* 1998; 57: 206-11.
[18] Kaufman DW, Kelly JP, Jurgelon JM, Anderson T, Issaragrisil S, Wiholm BE, et al. Drugs in the aetiology of agranulocytosis and aplastic anaemia. *Eur. J. Haematol.* 1996; 60 (Suppl): 23-30.
[19] Kelly JP, Kaufman DW, Shapiro S. Risks of agranulocytosis and aplastic anemia in relation to the use of cardiovascular drugs: The International Agranulocytosis and Aplastic Anemia Study. *Clin. Pharmacol. Ther.* 1991; 49: 330-41.
[20] Andrès E, Maloisel F. Idiosyncratic drug-induced agranulocytosis or acute neutropenia. *Curr. Opinion. Hematol.* 2008; 15: 15-21.
[21] Julia A, Olona M, Bueno J, Revilla E, Rosselo J, Petit J et al. Drug-induced agranulocytosis: prognostic factors in a series of 168 episodes. *Br. J. Hematol.* 1991; 79: 366-72.
[22] Andrès E, Kurtz JE, Martin-Hunyadi C, Kaltenbach G, Alt M, Weber JC, et al. Non-chemotherapy drug-induced agranulocytosis in elderly patients: the effects of Granulocyte Colony-Stimulating Factor. *Am. J. Med.* 2002; 112: 460-4.
[23] Andrès E, Noel E, Kurtz JE, Henoun Loukili N, Kaltenbach G, Maloisel F. Life-threatening idiosyncratic drug-induced agranulocytosis in elderly patients. *Drugs Aging* 2004; 21: 427-35.
[24] Tajiri J, Noguchi S, Murakami T, Murakami N. Antithyroid drug-induced agranulocytosis. The usefulness of routine white blood cell count monitoring. *Arch. Intern. Med.* 1990; 150: 621-4.

[25] Tajiri J. Antithyroid drug-induced agranulocytosis: special reference to normal white cell count agranulocytosis. *Thyroid* 2004; 14: 459-62.
[26] Maloisel F, Andrès E, Kaltenbach G, Noel E, Martin-Hunyadi C, Dufour P. Prognostic factors of hematological recovery in life-threatening nonchemotherapy drug-induced agranulocytosis. A study of 91 patients from a single center. *Presse. Med.* 2004; 33: 1164-8.
[27] Carey PJ. Drug-induced myelosuppression : diagnosis and management. *Drug Safety* 2003; 26: 691-706.
[28] Andrès E, Kurtz JE, Perrin AE, Dufour P, Schlienger JL, Maloisel F. The use of haematopoietic growth factors in antithyroid-related drug-induced agranulocytosis: a report of 20 patients. *Q. J. Med.* 2001; 94: 423-8.
[29] Sprikkelman A, de Wolf JTM, Vellenga E. Application of haematopoietic growth factors in drug-induced agranulocytosis: a review of 70 cases. *Leukemia* 1994; 8: 2031-6.
[30] Beauchesne MF, Shalansky SJ. Nonchemotherapy drug-induced agranulocytosis: a review of 118 patients treated with colony-stimulating factors. *Pharmacotherapy* 1999; 19: 299-305.
[31] Ibáñez L, Sabaté M, Ballarín E, Puig R, Vidal X, Laporte JR *et al.* Use of granulocyte colony-stimulating factor (G-CSF) and outcome in patients with non-chemotherapy agranulocytosis. *Pharmacoepidemiol Drug Saf.* 2008 Jan 8 [Epub ahead of print].
[32] Andrès E, Maloisel F, Zimmer J. The role of haematopoietic growth factors G-CSF and GM-CSF in the management of drug-induced agranulocytosis. *Br. J. Haematol.* 2010; 150: 3-8.
[33] Fukata S, Kuma K, Sugawara M. Granulocyte colony-stimulating factor (G-CSF) does not improve recovery from antithyroid drug-induced agranulocytosis: a prospective study. *Thyroïd* 1999; 9: 29-31.
[34] Bhatt V, Saleem A. Drug-induced neutropenia: pathophysiology, clinical features, and management. *Ann. Clin. Lab. Sci.* 2004; 34: 131-7.
[35] Andrès E, Noel E, Maloisel F. Long-term outcome of patients treated with hematopoietic growth factors for idiosyncratic drug-induced agranulocytosis. *Am. J. Med.* 2004; 116: 354.

In: Septic Shock
Editors: M. Johnston and J. Knight

ISBN: 978-1-62257-485-8
© 2012 Nova Science Publishers, Inc.

Chapter 5

SEPSIS: A DISEASE OF THE MICROCIRCULATION

*Farid Sadaka**
Critical Care Medicine / NeuroCritical Care
Medical Director, Trauma and Neuro ICU
Mercy Hospital St Louis / St. Louis University Hospital
St. Louis, MO, US

ABSTRACT

Regional tissue distress caused by microcirculatory dysfunction underlies the parthophysiology in sepsis. Despite correction of systemic oxygen delivery variables and macrocirculatory variables, regional hypoxia and oxygen extraction deficit persist. The microcirculation consists of the smallest blood vessels (<100 μm diameter) where oxygen release to the tissues takes place, and consists of arterioles, capillaries, and venules. The recent development of new medical imaging techniques, used in clinical investigations, has helped to identify the microcirculation as playing a key role in sepsis. Sepsis affects almost every cellular component of the microcirculation, including endothelial cells, smooth muscle cells, leukocytes, erythrocytes, and tissue cells. If not corrected directly, a poorly functioning microvasculature can lead to respiratory distress in tissue cells further fuelling microcirculatory dysfunction in a cascade of pathogenic mechanisms leading to organ failure.

---

* Fax: 314-251-4155. Phone: 314-251-6486; farid.sadaka@mercy.net

Endothelial cells seem to play a central role in coordinating the microcirculatory system and promoting tissue perfusion and oxygen supply. In a pathologic situation such as sepsis, abnormal interendothelial cell coupling and an abnormal arteriolar conducted response may account for impaired tissue perfusion and abnormal oxygen extraction. Microcirculatory distress is the single independent factor predicting outcome of septic patients. In the shunting theory of sepsis, the origin of oxygen extraction deficit in sepsis is due to oxygen transport being shunted to the venous compartment past dysfunctioning and collapsed microcirculatory units. In this theory the collapse of weak microcirculatory units may result in oxygen transport being shunted past the microcirculation resulting in regional ischemia and manifesting itself as a defect in oxygen extraction. Microcirculatory dysfunction persisting for extended periods of time can act as a motor driving the pathogenic effects of sepsis.

In humans, and especially in critically ill patients, the evaluation of the microcirculation has long been difficult. Recent years have witnessed the development of new techniques that can either directly visualize or indirectly evaluate microvascular perfusion and flow. Microvideoscopic techniques, such as orthogonal polarization spectral (OPS) and sidestream dark field (SDF) imaging, directly evaluate microvascular networks covered by a thin epithelium, such as the sublingual microcirculation. Laser Doppler and tissue O2 measurements detect global decreases in tissue perfusion but not heterogeneity of microvascular perfusion. These techniques may help to evaluate the dynamic response of the microcirculation to a stress test. In patients with severe sepsis and septic shock, the microcirculation is characterized by a decrease in capillary density and in the proportion of perfused capillaries, together with a blunted response to a vascular occlusion test. Guiding resuscitation with the use of these tools may allow more complete resuscitation and improve outcomes of patients with sepsis. I will thus discuss possible implications for the treatment of septic patients with interventions aimed to recruit and open the microcirculation.

INTRODUCTION

In the United States alone, approximately 750,000 cases of sepsis occur each year, of which at least 225,000 are fatal. One study evaluating the epidemiology of sepsis between 1979 and 2000 demonstrated an 8.7% increase in the annual incidence of sepsis. The cost of management of one septic patient has been estimated at $50,000, amounting to annual costs of approximately $17 billion. Sepsis is the leading cause of death in non-coronary

Intensive Care Units (ICUs), and the tenth leading cause of death overall. Organ failure occurs in about one third of patients with sepsis and severe sepsis is associated with an estimated mortality rate of 30-50%. Seventy percent of patients with three or more organ failures (classified as severe sepsis or septic shock) die [1-9]. The measurement of global hemodynamics reflects only a tiny part of whole-body circulatory blood flow. The microcirculation, with its huge endothelial surface, is in fact the largest 'organ' in the human body.

MICROCIRCULATION

Microcirculatory function is the main prerequisite for adequate tissue oxygenation and thus organ function. Its main role is to transport oxygen and nutrients to tissue cells, and maintain adequate immunological function. In disease, it serves to deliver therapeutic drugs to target cells. The microcirculation consists of the smallest blood vessels (<100 μm diameter) where oxygen release to the tissues takes place, and consists of arterioles, capillaries, and venules. The main cell types comprising the microcirculation are the endothelial cells lining the inside of the microvessels, smooth muscle cells (mostly in arterioles), red blood cells, leukocytes, and plasma components in blood [10].

The endothelium lining the inside of the microvessels plays a central role in function of the microcirculation by sensing flow, metabolic, and other regulating substances and regulating arteriolar smooth-muscle-cell tone and capillary recruitment. The endothelium is composed of a single layer of cells that lines the interior surface of all blood vessels. It is estimated to comprise around 10^{13} cells, weigh 1.5 kg and cover 4,000–7,000 m2, equivalent to six football fields. Endothelial cells are highly influenced by their environment [11, 12]. They can rapidly modulate their structure and function in response to chemical or physical stimuli, such as a change in blood flow. The endothelium plays a role in primary hemostasis, coagulation, fibrinolysis, immunity and regulation of vasomotor tone. During sepsis, most endothelial functions are disrupted, leading to a procoagulant, antifibrinolytic and proadhesive state [13]. The endothelium and smooth muscle of arteries and arterioles seem to be coupled both structurally and functionally. Sensing involves local depolarization and hyperpolarization of the capillary endothelial cell, and communication is achieved by an electronic spread via endothelium–smooth muscle cell-to-cell gap junctions. In a pathologic situation such as sepsis, abnormal interendothelial cell coupling and an abnormal arteriolar conducted response may account for impaired tissue perfusion and abnormal oxygen extraction [14].

THE SHUNTING THEORY OF SEPSIS

In sepsis and septic shock, the microcirculation is severely compromised because of an increased number of activated neutrophils with decreased deformability and increased aggregability, upregulation of adhesion molecules, decreased deformability of red blood cells, activation of the clotting cascade with fibrin deposition and the formation of microthrombi, dysfunction of vascular autoregulatory mechanisms, as well as enhanced perfusion of large arteriovenous shunts [15-19]. These processes together lead to the shut-down of vulnerable microcirculatory units in the organ beds, promoting the shunting of oxygen transport from the arterial to the venous compartment leaving the microcirculation hypoxic. In this so-called shunting theory of sepsis, adequate oxygen delivery is not successful in delivering oxygen to weak shunted microcirculatory units [20]. This results in an oxygen extraction deficit of these shunted units with raised levels of venous pO2 and lactate with apparent sufficient oxygen delivery (Figure 1).

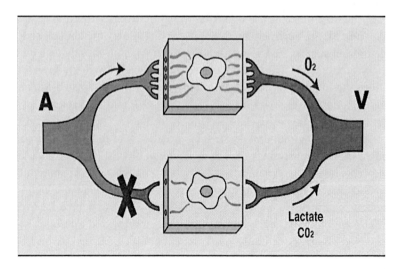

Figure 1. Shunting Theory of Sepsis.

As a result, the microcirculatory partial pressure of O2 (μpO2) drops below the venous pO2; the difference between the two has been termed the "pO2 gap", a measurement of the severity of functional shunting [21, 22].

This explains why systemic hemodynamic-derived and oxygen-derived variables are not able to sense such microcirculatory distress and thus mask this pathophysiologic process ongoing in sepsis and septic shock [10]. The result is microcirculatory dysfunction despite the correction of systemic hemodynamic- and oxygen-derived variables. In sepsis and septic shock, all three elements of the microvascular network are compromised, namely arteriolar hyporesponsiveness, a reduced number of perfused capillaries, and venular obstruction by the sequestration of activated neutrophils [23].

MONITORING THE MICROCIRCULATION

'Downstream' global derivatives of microcirculatory dysfunction such as lactate, tonometry, mixed venous oxygen saturation (SvO2) or central venous oxygen saturation (ScvO2), and measurements of Oxygen delivery (DO2) and oxygen uptake/consumption (VO2), are used in daily clinical management of severe septic and septic shock patients. Lactate levels are thought to reflect anaerobic metabolism associated with tissue dysoxia and are measured in order to monitor response to therapy and for prognosis [24]. It is difficult to interpret lactate levels, since they are dependant on the balance between lactate production due to global , regional , and cellular (mitochondrial dysfunction) factors on the one hand, and lactate clearance depending on adequate liver function on the other hand [25]. SvO2 and ScvO2 are thought to reflect the average oxygen saturation of all perfused microvascular beds. In sepsis, microcirculatory shunting can cause normal SvO2/ScvO2 in the presence of severe local tissue dysoxia [21]. Fiddian-Green and Baker introduced regional intestinal capnography as a means to evaluate tissue dysoxia [26]. This progressed to include CO2 measurements for sublingual, buccal, and subcutaneous microcirculatory CO2 levels [27-30]. In sepsis however, the interpretation of tonometric results is affected by microcirculatory shunting, since areas with reduced perfusion and CO2 offloading are next to hypoxic regions [31]. Most importantly, all these parameters are indirect and downstream from the pathological processes taking place in the microcirculatory beds. Direct assessment of the microcirculation would be the more superior and preferred method. Intravital microscopy (IVM) is one of the earliest technologies used in animals in vivo. In humans, IVM studies are restricted to the eye, the skin and the nail fold owing to the size of the IVM equipment and the use of fluorescent dyes for contrast enhancement. Observations with IVM are limited to superficial layers of thin tissues only, with improved contrast by using fluorescent dyes. Because of the potentially toxic effects of these dyes in humans, studies are mostly limited to animals [32, 33].

NAILFOLD VIDEOCAPILLAROSCOPY

Nailfold microvideoscopy (Table 1) was the first method used at the bedside.

Table 1. Summary of techniques for the quantification of microcirculatory variables in humans

Technique	Variable measured	Area studied	Remarks/Limitations
Nailfold micro-videoscopy	Vascular density, heterogeneity, flow	Fingers	sensitive to changes in temperature and peripheral vasoconstriction; mainly used to study the microvasculature in chronic illnesses
Laser Doppler	Flow (relative), hemoglobin content, microvascular reactivity test	Skin	measures flow in a variable volume of tissue and thus it is unable to detect it in individual vessels.
OPS and SDF	Vascular density, perfusion heterogeneity, flow	Sublingual, ostomy, skin, concunctiva, gingival, rectal mucosa	Semiquantitative, motion artifacts, need for manual intervention
NIRS	Tissue O2 saturation (StO2), Vaso-occlusive test (VOT)	Thenar eminence	Global measurement in sampled volume (mixture of arterioles, capillaries, and venules), VOT is more useful than StO2 in sepsis

NIRS = Near-infrared spectroscopy; OPS = Orthogonal Polarization Spectral; SDF = Sidestream Dark Field.

The junction between cuticle and nail is coated with transparent oil and placed on the stage of an ordinary microscope. This area is sensitive to changes in temperature and peripheral vasoconstriction that happens during septic shock and vasopressor use [34]. Therefore, this technique is mainly used to study the microvasculature in chronic illnesses, like diabetes, and not in critically ill septic shock patients.

LASER DOPPLER

Laser Doppler (Table 1) can be used to measure microvascular blood flow in an area between 0.5 and 1 mm^3, so that the flow measured represents flow in at least 50 vessels, including arterioles, capillaries, and venules of variable size, direction, and perfusion [35]. Therefore, the main limitation of this technique is that it measures flow in a variable volume of tissue and thus it is unable to detect it in individual vessels. Some laser doppler devices do allow a test of vasoreactivity. A cuff is placed around the arm, and then rapidly released. The ascending slope after this occlusion is relieved is used as a marker of endothelial reactivity, and thus a surrogate for the functional integrity and health of the microcirculation [36]. This device can currently only be applied in humans to study skin microvasculature [37].

ORTHOGONAL POLARIZATION SPECTRAL AND SIDESTREAM DARK FIELD IMAGING

In Orthogonal polarization spectral (OPS) imaging (Table 1), the tissue embedding the microcirculation is illuminated with polarized green light [38]. Backscattered (and thus depolarized) light is projected onto a camera after it passes an analyzer.

The light reflected by the tissue surface is blocked by this analyzer. By elimination of the reflected light and imaging of only the backscattered light, subsurface structures, such as the microcirculation, can be observed. The use of green light ensures sufficient optical absorption by the (de)oxyhemoglobin-containing red blood cells (RBCs) with respect to the lack of absorption by the tissue embedding the microcirculation, creating contrast (i.e., RBCs are visualized black and tissue is visualized white/grayish). OPS has several limitations; suboptimal imaging of the capillaries due to motion-induced image blurring. Also in larger vessels, especially during continuous flow, it is difficult to observe the granular nature of flowing blood cells due to blurring of images. As a result, a newer version based on the same principals was developed; Sidestream Dark Field (SDF) imaging (Table 1). In SDF imaging, illumination is provided by surrounding a central light guide by concentrically placed light emitting diodes (LEDs) to provide sidestream dark field illumination (Figure 2).

The lens system in the core of the light guide is optically isolated from the illuminating outer ring thus preventing the microcirculatory image from contamination by tissue surface reflections. Light from the illuminating outer core of the SDF probe, which penetrates the tissue illuminates the tissue-embedded microcirculation by scattering. The LEDs emit at a central wavelength of 530 nm, to ensure optimal optical absorption by the hemoglobin in the RBCs, independent of its oxygenation state. This leads to an image where RBCs are imaged as dark moving globules against a white/grayish background. To improve the imaging of moving structures such as flowing RBCs, the LEDs provide pulsed illumination in synchrony with the camera frame rate to perform intravital stroboscopy. This stroboscopic imaging prevents smearing of moving features, such as flowing RBCs, and motion-induced blurring of capillaries due to the short illumination intervals [38].

These techniques can be used only on organs covered by a thin epithelial layer. In humans, they can be applied to the skin, conjunctiva, gingiva, sublingual area, ileostomies or colostomies, and rectal mucosa.

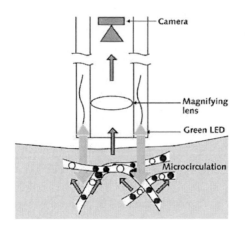
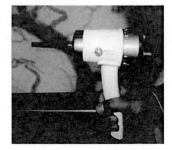

Figure 2. SDF: Sidestream Dark Field.

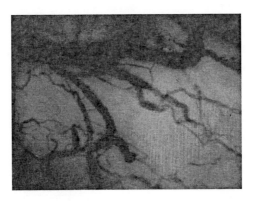

Figure 3. A still image of the human sublingual microcirculation as visualized by sidestrem dark field (SDF) microscopy.

The sublingual microcirculation has been the most extensively studied in patients with critical illness and sepsis. Capillaries and venules of variable size can be visualized; arterioles are usually not visualized because they are located in deeper layers. Video images (Figure 3) are captured with the handheld device. After the removal of saliva and other secretions using gauze, the device is gently applied (without significant pressure) to the lateral side of the tongue, in an area approximately 1.5–4 cm from the tip of the tongue.

Video recordings of 20-30 seconds in duration are analyzed using specific softwares, however, manual intervention is still needed for vessel identification as well as for blood flow measurement.

Different variables can be measured, including vascular density, heterogeneity of perfusion, and microvascular blood flow. These are usually measured using a semiquantitative analysis, which can easily be performed by experienced investigators, with excellent reliability (intra- and interobserver variabilities within 5–10% [39] and excellent agreement between investigators [40]. The main limitations of these techniques are secretions and motion artifacts that may impair image quality. They are only feasible in sedated or cooperative patients. The need for manual intervention is also a limitation of these techniques.

NEAR-INFRARED SPECTROSCOPY

Near-infrared spectroscopy (NIRS) (Table 1) is a technique that utilizes near-infrared light to measure chromophores (oxy- and deoxyhemoglobin, myoglobin, and cytochrome aa3) in tissues [41]. The fractions of oxy- and deoxyhemoglobin are used to calculate tissue O2 saturation (StO2). In addition, total light absorption is used to compute total tissue hemoglobin (HbT) and the absolute tissue hemoglobin index (THI), two indicators of blood volume in the region of microvasculature sensed by the probe [41, 42]. The thenar eminence has been used in most studies using NIRS because the thickness of skin and adipose tissue covering this muscle is less influenced by edema, or body mass index [43] (Figure 4 A).

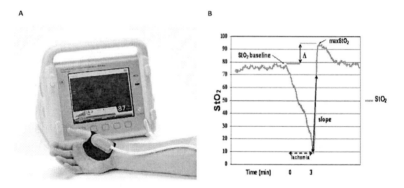

Figure 4. A. Near-infrared spectroscopy. B. Vaso-occlusive test by NIRS.

The analysis of changes in StO2 during a brief episode of forearm ischemia (Vaso occlusive test [VOT]) enables quantification of microvascular dysfunction. The downslope during the VOT is suggestive of oxygen consumption of the muscle tissue and the upslope after relieve of the ischemia is suggestive of the microcirculatory recruitment and health (Figure 4 B). This technique has its limitations. NIRS signal is limited to vessels that have a diameter less than 1 mm (arterioles, capillaries, and venules), and thus represents the aggregate of O2 saturations in the sampling volume. In addition, NIRS does not measure microcirculatory blood flow.

THE MICROCIRCULATION IN SEPSIS

Sepsis and Outcome

Using OPS and SDF devices, investigators have reported that the microcirculation is markedly altered in sepsis, that alterations are more severe in nonsurvivors, and that persistent microvascular alterations are associated with development of multiple organ failure and death [39, 44, 45]. Using NIRS, investigators have shown that oxygen consumption and microvascular reactivity (during stagnant ischemia, VOT) are altered in sepsis, are more severe in nonsurvivors, and persistence is associated with development of multiple organ failure and death [46-49]. In all these studies, microcirculatory alterations were similar during the initial 24 hrs of shock, but the persistence of these alterations was associated with the development of multiorgan failure (MOF) and death. An important finding was that microcirculatory alterations, but not the global hemodynamic or oxygenation variables, were related to the occurrence and the severity of MOF and death. Global hemodynamic and oxygenation variables were similar despite the significantly altered microcirculation in nonsurvivors. Compared to changes in heart rate, mean arterial blood pressure, central venous pressure, pulmonary artery occlusion pressure, cardiac index, SvO_2, DO_2, VO_2, lactate levels, and SOFA score, the changes in small vessel perfusion as determined by OPS between the first and second day of shock as well as between the first and last day of shock were more sensitive and specific predictors of outcomes [45].

VASOPRESSORS AND INOTROPES

Norepinephrine

Norepinephrine (Table 2) is the most commonly used and advocated vasopressor in septic shock to maintain MAP > 65 mmHg. In one study, norepinephrine administration aimed at achieving a MAP above 65 mmHg (54 mmHg to 77 mmHg) in septic shock patients with life threatening hypotension resulted in improvement of NIRS variables measured at the level of the thenar eminence [50]. Using SDF, Jhanji et al [51] showed that increasing MAP from 60 to 70, 80, and 90 mm Hg by increasing the norepinephrine dose had no significant effect on the microcirculation. Using the same SDF imaging techniques and a similar protocol with MAP at 65, 75, and 85 mm Hg, Dubin and colleagues [52] reported no change in the sublingual microcirculation. However, Thooft et al, using both SDF and NIRS, showed that increasing MAP from 65 to 75 to 85 resulted in increased cardiac output, improved microcirculatory function, and decreased lactate concentrations [53]. In all these studies, the microvascular response was variable between patients. This suggests that individualization of blood pressure targets may be warranted.

Dobutamine

Dobutamine (predominantly b2-adrenergic) has both inotropic and vasodilatory effects (Table 2), and is advocated as part of the early-goal directed therapy of eligible patients with severe sepsis and septic shock [54]. In one study, the addition of dobutamine in septic patients was associated with improved OPS-measured sublingual microcirculatory perfusion over time, irrespective of changes in systemic hemodynamic variables [55]. This suggests a role of dobutamine in microcirculatory recruitment in septic patients that is separate from its role in improving oxygen and hemodynamic variables.

Levosimendan

Levosimendan (calcium sensitizer) improves cardiac contractility and has a mild vasodilatory effect (Table 2). In a prospective study using SDF, Morelli et al showed that Levosimendan, compared to dobutamine, improved sublingual microcirculatory blood flow in volume resuscitated patients with septic shock. This effect did not correlate with changes in systemic hemodynamics and flow variables [56]. These findings strengthen the assumption that levosimendan similar to dobutamine – by its vasodilatory effects – improves microcirculatory blood flow by increasing the driving pressure of blood flow at the entrance of the microcirculation, irrespective of its the effects on myocardial contractility.

Vasodilators

In one report using OPS, eight patients responded to an intravenous bolus of 0.5 mg Nitroglycerin (NTG) after adequate resuscitation with a significant increase in sublingual microcirculatory variables [57]. However, in a double-blind placebo-controlled setting, in adequately resuscitated severe septic and septic shock patients, sublingual microcrocirculatory variables were not different from placebo [58]. The role of vasodilators in sepsis as a therapeutic strategy to recruit the microcirculation remains controversial and is yet to be elucidated (Table 2).

Table 2. Interventions in sepsis (summary of effects in human studies on microcirculatory variables)

Intervention	Technique (s)	Effects	Remarks	References
Norepinephrine (NE)	NIRS	Improved	NE used to achieve MAP>65	[50]
Norepinephrine (NE)	SDF	No effect	NE used to increase MAP from 60 to 70 to 80 to 90 mmHg	[51]
Norepinephrine (NE)	SDF	No effect	NE used to increase MAP from 65 to 75 to 85mmHg	[52]
Norepinephrine (NE)	NIRS and SDF	Improved	NE used to increase MAP from 65 to 75 to 85mmHg	[53]
Dobutamine	OPS	Improved	irrespective of changes in systemic hemodynamic variables	[55]
Levosimendan	SDF	Improved	Compared to Dobutamine;irrespective of changes in systemic hemodynamic variables	[56]
Nitroglycerin	OPS	Improved	8 patients, observational study	[57]
Nitroglycerin	SDF	No effect	double-blind placebo-controlled setting	[58]
Red blood cell transfusion (Leukoreduced)	NIRS (62) SDF (63)	No effect	Improved in patients with altered microcirculation at baseline	[62, 63]
Red blood cell transfusion (non-leukoreduced)	NIRS and SDF	No effect	muscle oxygen consumption improved in patients with low baseline and deteriorated in patients with preserved baseline	[64]
Lactate Ringer and Albumin	SDF	Improved	Both fluids improved microcirculation in early (within 24 hrs) and not late after 48 hrs); independent of hemodynamics and type of fluid.	[67]
Hydrocortisone	OPS	improved	not influenced by the response to an ACTH test	[70]

NIRS = Near-infrared spectroscopy; OPS = Orthogonal Polarization Spectral; SDF = Sidestream Dark Field.

Red Blood Cell Transfusion

Red blood cell transfusion is one of the most commonly used interventions in the ICU to treat severe anemia, which often occurs in sepsis. In the United States, more than14 million units of packed red blood cells (RBCs) are administered annually, many of which are administered in the ICU [59].

Approximately 40 to 80% of RBC transfusions in the ICU are not given for bleeding, but rather for low hemoglobin levels, for a decrease in physiological reserve, or for alterations in tissue perfusion [60,61]. In addition, RBC transfusion is recommended as part of early goal-directed therapy for patients with severe sepsis and septic shock [54].

In a general critically ill population, using NIRS, muscle tissue oxygenation, oxygen consumption and microvascular reactivity were globally unaltered by leukoreduced RBC transfusion in a study by Creteur et al [62]. However, muscle oxygen consumption and microvascular reactivity improved following transfusion in patients with alterations of these variables at baseline [62]. In severe septic patient requiring leukoreduced RBC transfusion, using SDF, Sakr et al showed that the sublingual microcirculation was globally unaltered , however, it improved in patients with altered capillary perfusion at baseline [63].

Using both SDF and NIRS, Sadaka et al looked at patients that got non-leukoreduced RBCs for a hemoglobin <7.0, or for a hemoglobin between 7.0 and 9.0 with either lactic acidosis or central venous oxygen saturation < 70% [64].

Sadaka et al showed that muscle tissue oxygen consumption, microvascular reactivity, and sublingual microcirculation were globally unaltered by RBC transfusion in severe septic patients. However, muscle oxygen consumption improved in patients with low baseline and deteriorated in patients with preserved baseline [64]. Future research with larger samples is needed to further examine the association between RBC transfusion and outcomes of patients resuscitated early in severe sepsis, with an emphasis on elucidating the potential contribution of microvascular factors. (Table 2).

Fluids

Early, effective fluid resuscitation is a key component in the management of patients with severe sepsis and septic shock with the goal of improving tissue perfusion. Optimizing tissue perfusion is proven to improve outcome in this patient population [65], is standard of care and a crucial part of the surviving sepsis campaign [54]. The best fluid in this early resuscitation phase has and still is under debate.

Several experimental studies have also shown that fluids may improve the microcirculation in sepsis. Interestingly, Hoffman et al. showed that hydroxyethyl starch (HES 130 kD) but not saline solutions improved functional capillary density in hamster skinfold [66]. In a recent clinical trial to evaluate the differential effect of crystalloid (Lactate Ringer) vs Colloid (4% Albumin), De Backer et al found that fluid administration improved microvascular perfusion in the early (within 24 hrs) but not late (after 48 hrs) phase of sepsis [67].

This effect was independent of global hemodynamic effects and of the type of solution. Considering the importance of fluid resuscitation in severe sepsis/septic shock, and the importance of the microcirculation in the pathophysiology and as therapeutic target in this patient population, it is warranted to study the effects of different fluids on the microcirculation.

In an ongoing study, Sadaka et al is evaluating the effect of different fluids (Albumin 5%, Normal Saline, HES 130 kD) on the microcirculation in the first 24 hrs of resuscitation of severe sepsis/septic shock patients [68].(Table 2).

Steroids

Moderate doses of corticosteroids have been advocated as part of the management of patients with septic shock [54], even though the outcome benefit of this strategy has recently been challenged [69].

The mechanisms for possible microcirculatory improvement could be attributed to restoration of vascular responsiveness to catecholamines in septic shock thus leading to an increase in perfusion pressure, anti-inflammatory properties of steroids, and modulation of nitric oxide (NO) production.

Using OPS, Bu¨chele et al showed that the administration of moderate doses of hydrocortisone in early septic shock resulted in a modest but consistent improvement in capillary perfusion [70]. The improvement was seen already in the first hour after administration of hydrocortisone and was not influenced by the response to an ACTH test [70]. However, further studies are needed to elucidate the effect of steroids and the mechanisms of steroids effect on the microcirculation. (Table 2)

Sedatives

Sedation is widely used in critically ill patients, however, adverse effects of sedation have not been fully evaluated, especially in septic shock patients. Using laser Doppler flowmetry, in a group of nonseptic patients, Lamblin et al showed that sedation with midazolam or a combination of midazolam and sufentanil induced a deterioration of vasomotion and microvascular response to ischaemia [71]. In another group of nonseptic patients, using OPS, Koch et al showed that a short-term infusion of propofol reduced microcirculatory perfusion [72]. In another study of propofol, using SDF, Jung et al didn't document any effect of propofol on the microcirculation in hemodynamically stable intensive care unit patients [73]. The effect of sedatives on the microcirculation of septic and septic shock patients needs to be elucidated.

CONCLUSION

There is a shift of research focus from global hemodynamic parameters to microcirculation monitoring in sepsis. The microcirculation may actually prove to be a logical next frontier in understanding the full scope of organ failure and mortality in septic shock patients. Although clinical investigations and recent guidelines in sepsis management have traditionally focused on macrocirculatory hemodynamics that reflect the distribution of blood flow globally throughout the body, a functional microcirculation is a critical component of the cardiovascular system that is necessary for effective blood flow and delivery of vital nutrients and therapies to tissues. With the advent of new technologies, it is now possible to visualize the microcirculation in human subjects at the bedside. In septic patients, microcirculatory failure appears to be of major prognostic significance. Abnormal microcirculation in the early resuscitation phase as well as the persistence of microcirculatory derangements over time, have been associated with lower survival in septic shock patients.

A lack of improvement in microcirculatory variables early in the course has been associated with multiorgan failure and death, thus pointing to the time-sensitive impact of the microcirculation and the possibility that the microcirculation needs to be an early therapeutic target. Therapeutic approaches to counteract microcirculatory failure could represent a novel strategy to help optimize tissue perfusion in sepsis resuscitation. There are some important limitations to studying the microcirculation in septic patients.

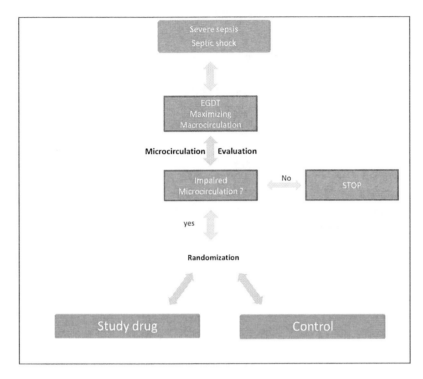

Figure 5. A template for designing a randomized clinical trial of a novel agent to recruit the microcirculation and possibly improve outcome in severe sepsis and septic shock. (EGDT = Early-goal Directed Therapy).

One limitation is the need for technologies that one can use to get full quantitative rather than semiquantitative measurements of the microcirculatory variables. In addition, these technologies need to provide real-time readouts at the bedside, so they can be used clinically to evaluate resuscitative efforts of the microcirculation, and not simply for research purposes by experienced investigators. Furthermore, the microcirculation needs to be studied in conjuction with other possible players in multiorgan failure and death. A very important player is the mitochondria. Whether the primary cause of oxygen extraction deficit in sepsis is the presence of shunted weak microcirculatory units or diseased mitochondria unable to process oxygen remains a matter of dispute [74, 75]. Resuscitation of the circulatory failure associated with sepsis based on correcting systemic hemodynamic- and oxygen-derived variables, but where regional and microcirculatory distress persist, has been termed microcirculatory and mitochondrial distress syndrome (MMDS) [10, 76]. An ideal agent in the therapy of MMDS in sepsis would most likely target 1) the endothelium, 2) the arterioles in order to recruit low-flow microcirculatory units, 3) the mitochondria or 4) a combination of the above. Figure 5 shows a template for a randomized clinical trial of a novel microcirculation-directed therapy in severe sepsis and septic shock for future trials. Such a trial would require a real-time assessment of the microcirculation prior to decision to randomize (Figure 5).

REFERENCES

[1] Martin, GS; Mannino, DM; Eaton, S; Moss, M. The epidemiology of sepsis in the United States from 1979 through 2000. *N Engl J Med,* 2003 348 (16), 1546-54.

[2] Brun-Buisson, C; Doyon, F; Carlet, J. Incidence, risk factors, and outcome of severe sepsis and septic shock in adults: a multicenter prospective study in intensive care units. *JAMA,* 1995 274, 968-74.

[3] Karlsson, S; Ruokonen, E; Varpula, T; Ala-Kokko, TI; Pettilä, V.; Finnsepsis Study Group. Longterm outcome and quality-adjusted life years after severe sepsis. *Crit. Care Med,* 2009 37, 1268- 74.

[4] Angus, DC; Linde-Zwirble, WT; Lidicker, J; Clermont, G; Carcillo, J; Pinsky, MR. Epidemiology of severe sepsis in the United States: analysis of incidence, outcome, and associated costs of care. *Crit Care Med,* 2001 29, 1303-1310.

[5] Chalfin, DB; Holbein, ME; Fein, AM; Carlon, GC. Cost-effectiveness of monoclonal antibodies to gram-negative endotoxin in the treatment of gram-negative sepsis in ICU patients. *JAMA,* 1993 269, 249-254.

[6] Wheeler, AP; Bernard, GR. Treating patients with severe sepsis. *N. Engl. J. Med,* 1999 340, 207-214.

[7] Parrillo, JE; Parker, MM; Natanson, C; Suffredini, AF; Danner, RL; Cunnion, RE; Ognibene FP. Septic shock in humans: advances in the understanding of pathogenesis, cardiovascular dysfunction, and therapy. *Ann. Intern. Med,* 1990 113, 227-242.

[8] Angus, DC; Wax, RS. Epidemiology of sepsis: an update. *Crit. Care Med,.* 2001 29(Suppl 7), S109-16.

[9] Sands, KE; Bates, DW; Lanken, PN; Graman, PS; Hibberd, PL; Kahn, KL; Parsonnet, J; Panzer, R; Orav, EJ; Snydman, DR; Black, E; Schwartz, JS; Moore, R; Johnson, BL Jr; Platt, R; Academic Medical Center Consortium Sepsis Project Working Group. Epidemiology of

sepsis syndrome in 8 academic medical centers. *JAMA,* 1997 278(3), 234-40.
[10] Ince, C. The microcirculation is the motor of sepsis. *Critical Care,* 2005 9(suppl 4), S13-S19.
[11] Augustin, HG; Kozian, DH; Johnson, RC. Differentiation of endothelial cells: analysis of the constitutive and activated endothelial cell phenotypes. *Bioessays,* 1994 16, 901– 906.
[12] Wolinsky, H; Katz, D; Markle, R; Mills, J; Brem, S; Wassertheil-Smoller, S. Hydrolase activities in the rat aorta. IV. Relation between clearance rates of circulating 125I-labeled lowdensity lipoproteins and levels of tissue hydrolase activity. *Circ. Res,* 1980 47, 433–442.
[13] Ait-Oufella, H; Maury, E; Lehoux, S; Guidet, B; Offenstadt, G. The endothelium: physiological functions and role in microcirculatory failure during severe sepsis. *Intensive Care Med,* 2010 36(8), 1286-98.
[14] Vallet, B. Endothelial cell dysfunction and abnormal tissue perfusion. *Crit Care Med,* 2002 30(suppl 5), S229-S234.
[15] Avontuur, JA; Bruining, HA; Ince, C. Nitric oxide causes dysfunction of coronary autoregulation in endotoxemic rats. *Cardiovasc Res,* 1997 35, 368-376.
[16] Cronenwett, JL; Lindenauer, SM. Direct measurement of arteriovenous anastomotic blood flow in the septic canine hindlimb. *Surgery,* 1979 85,275-282.
[17] Astiz, ME; DeGent, GE; Lin, RY; Rackow, EC. Microvascular function and rheologic changes in hyperdynamic sepsis. *Crit. Care Med,* 1995 23, 265-271.
[18] Linderkamp, O; Ruef, P; Brenner, B; Gulbins, E; Lang, F. Passive deformability of mature, immature, and active neutrophils in healthy and septicemic neonates. *Pediatr Res.,* 1998 44, 946-950.
[19] Diaz, NL; Finol, HJ; Torres, SH; Zambrano, CI; Adjounian, H. Histochemical and ultrastructural study of skeletal muscle in patients with sepsis and multiple organ failure syndrome (MOFS). *Histol Histopathol,* 1998 13, 121-128.
[20] Buwalda, M; Ince, C. Opening the microcirculation: can vasodilators be useful in sepsis? *Intensive Care Med,* 2002 28(9), 1208-17.
[21] Ince, C; Sinaasappel, M. Microcirculatory oxygenation and shunting in sepsis and shock. *Crit .Care Med,* 1999 27, 1369-1377.
[22] Schwarte, LA; Fournell, A; van Bommel, J; Ince, C. Redistribution of intestinal microcirculatory oxygenation during acute hemodilution in pigs. *J. Appl. Physiol.,* 2005 98, 1070-1075.

[23] Lush, CW; Kvietys, PR. Microvascular dysfunction in sepsis. *Microcirculation*, 2000 7, 83-101.
[24] Bakker, J; Coffernils, M; Leon, M; Gris, P; Vincent, JL. Blood lactate levels are superior to oxygen-derived variables in predicting outcome in human septic shock. *Chest*, 1991 99, 956-962.
[25] De Backer D. Lactic acidosis. *Intensive Care Med*, 2003 29, 699- 702.
[26] Fiddian-Green, RG; Baker, S. Predictive value of the stomach wall pH for complications after cardiac operations: comparison with other monitoring. *Crit Care Med*, 1987 15, 153-156.
[27] Creteur, J; De Backer, D; Sakr, Y; Koch, M; Vincent, JL. Determinant of sublingual pCO2 in patients with septic shock. *Crit. Care Med. Suppl*, 2004 31, 419.
[28] Guzman, JA; Dikin, MS; Kruse, JA. Lingual, splanchnic, and systemic hemodynamic and carbon dioxide tension changes during endotoxic shock and resuscitation. *J. Appl. Physiol.*, 2005 98, 108-113.
[29] Weil, MH; Nakagawa, Y; Tang, W; Sato, Y; Ercoli, F; Finegan, R; Grayman, G; Bisera, J. Sublingual capnometry: a new noninvasive measurement for diagnosis and quantitation of severity of circulatory shock. *Crit Care Med*, 1999 27, 1225-1229.
[30] Venkatesh, B; Morgan, TJ; Hall, J; Willgoss, EZ. Subcutaneous gas tensions closely track ileal mucosal gas tensions in a model of endotoxemia without anaerobism. *Intensive Care Med.*, 2005 31, 447-454.
[31] Vallet, B; Ince, C. Noninvasive assessment of tissue oxygenation. *Semin Respir Crit. Care Med.*, 1999 20, 3-10.
[32] Saetzler, RK; Jallo, J; Lehr, HA; Philips, CM; Vasthare, U; Arfors, KE; Tuma, RF. Intravital fluorescence microscopy: impact of lightinduced phototoxicity on adhesion of fluorescently labeled leukocytes. *J. Histochem. Cytochem.*, 1997 45, 505-513.
[33] Steinbauer, M; Harris, AG; Abels, C; Messmer, K. Characterization and prevention of phototoxic effects in intravital fluorescence microscopy in the hamster dorsal skinfold model. *Langenbecks Arch. Surg*, 2000 385, 290-298.
[34] Awan, ZA; Wester, T; Kvernebo, K. Human microvascular imaging: a review of skin and tongue videomicroscopy techniques and analysing variables. *Clin. Physiol. Funct Imaging*, 2010 30, 79–88.
[35] De Backer, D; Ospina-Tascon, G; Salgado, D; Favory, R; Creteur, J; Vincent, JL. Monitoring the microcirculation in the critically ill patient:

current methods and future approaches. *Intensive Care Med.,* 2010 36(11), 1813-25.
[36] Lamblin, V; Favory, R; Boulo, M; Mathieu, D. Microcirculatory alterations induced by sedation in intensive care patients. Effects of midazolam alone and in association with sufentanil. *Crit. Care,* 2006 10, R176.
[37] Altintas, MA; Altintas, AA; Guggenheim, M; Steiert, AE; Aust, MC; Niederbichler, AD; Herold, C; Vogt, PM. Insight in human skin microcirculation using in vivo reflectance-mode confocal laser scanning microscopy. *J. Digit Imaging,* 2010 23(4), 475-81.
[38] Goedhart, PT; Khalilzada, M; Bezemer, R; Merza, J; Ince, C. Sidestream Dark Field (SDF) imaging: a novel stroboscopic LED ring-based imaging modality for clinical assessment of the microcirculation. *Opt. Express,* 2007 15(23), 15101-14.
[39] De Backer, D; Creteur, J; Preiser, JC; Dubois, MJ; Vincent, JL. Microvascular blood flow is altered in patients with sepsis. *Am. J. Respir. Crit Care Med,* 2002 166, 98–104.
[40] Boerma, EC; Mathura, KR; van der Voort, PH; Spronk, PE; Ince, C. Quantifying bedside-derived imaging of microcirculatory abnormalities in septic patients: a prospective validation 41- study. *Crit. Care,* 2005 9, R601–R606.
[41] Myers, DE; Anderson, LD; Seifert, RP; Ortner, JP; Cooper, CE; Beilman, GJ; Mowlem, JD. Noninvasive method for measuring local hemoglobin oxygen saturation in tissue using wide gap second derivative near-infrared spectroscopy. *J. Biomed. Opt,* 2005 10, 034017
[42] Creteur, J; Carollo, T; Soldati, G; Buchele, G; De Backer, D; Vincent JL. The prognostic value of muscle StO2 in septic patients. *Intensive Care Med.,* 2007 33, 1549–1556.
[43] Poeze, M. Tissue-oxygenation assessment using near-infrared spectroscopy during severe sepsis: confounding effects of tissue edema on StO2 values. *Intensive Care Med.,* 2006 32(5), 788-9.
[44] Trzeciak, S; Dellinger, RP; Parrillo, JE; Bajaj, J; Abate, NL; Arnold, RC; Colilla, S; Zanotti, S; Hollenberg, SM. Early microcirculatory perfusion derangements in patients with severe sepsis and septic shock: relationship to hemodynamics, oxygen transport, and survival. *Ann. Emerg. Med.,* 2007 49, 88-98.
[45] Sakr, Y; Dubois, MJ; De Backer, D; Creteur, J; Vincent, JL. Persistant microvasculatory alterations are associated with organ failure and death in patients with septic shock. *Crit. Care Med.,* 2004 32, 1825-1831.

[46] Doerschug, K; Delsing, A; Schmidt, G; Haynes, WG. Impairments in microvascular reactivity are related to organ failure in human sepsis. *Am J.Physiol. Heart Circ. Physiol.*, 2007 293, H1065–H1071.

[47] Pareznik, R; Knezevic, R; Voga, G; Podbregar, M. Changes in muscle tissue oxygenation during stagnant ischemia in septic patients. *Intensive Care Med.*, 2006 32, 87–92.

[48] Creteur, J; Carollo, T; Soldati, G; Buchele, G; De Backer, D; Vincent, JL. The prognostic value of muscle StO2 in septic patients. *Intensive Care Med.*, 2007 33, 1549–1556.

[49] Skarda, D; Mulier, K; Myers, D; Taylor, JH; Beilman, GJ. Dynamic Near-Infrared Spectroscopy Measurements in Patients with Severe Sepsis. *Shock,* 2007 27, 348-353.

[50] Georger, JF; Hamzaoui, O; Chaari, A; Maizel, J; Richard, C; Teboul, JL. Restoring arterial pressure with norepinephrine improves muscle tissue oxygenation assessed by near-infrared spectroscopy in severely hypotensive septic patients. *Intensive Care Med.,* 2010 36(11), 1882-9.

[51] Jhanji, S; Stirling, S; Patel, N; Hinds, CJ; Pearse, RM. The effect of increasing doses of norepinephrine on tissue oxygenation and microvascular flow in patients with septic shock. *Crit. Care Med.,* 2009 37, 1961-1966.

[52] Dubin, A; Pozo, MO; Casabella, CA; Palizas, F Jr; Murias, G; Moseinco, MC; Kanoore, E; Palizas, F; Estenssoro, E, Ince, C. Increasing arterial blood pressure with norepinephrine does not improve microcirculatory blood flow: a prospective study. *Crit. Care,* 2009 13, R92.

[53] Thooft, A; Favory, R; Salgado, DR; Taccone, FS; Donadello, K; De Backer, D; Creteur, J; Vincent, JL. Effects of changes in arterial pressure on organ perfusion during septic shock. *Crit .Care,* 2011 15(5), R222.

[54] Dellinger, RP; Levy, MM; Carlet, JM; Bion, J; Parker, MM; Jaeschke, R; Reinhart, K; Angus, DC; Brun-Buisson, C; Beale, R; Calandra, T; Dhainaut, JF; Gerlach, H; Harvey, M; Marini, JJ; Marshall, J; Ranieri, M; Ramsay, G; Sevransky, J; Thompson, BT; Townsend, S; Vender, JS; Zimmerman, JL; Vincent, JL. Surviving Sepsis Campaign: International guidelines for management of severe sepsis and septic shock: 2008 [published correction appears in *Crit. Care Med.* 2008; 36:1394-1396]. *Crit Care Med,* 2008 36, 296-327.

[55] De Backer, D; Creteur, J; Dubois, MJ; Sakr, Y; Koch, M; Verdant, C; Vincent, JL. The effects of dobutamine on microcirculatory alterations

in patients with septic shock are independent of its systemic effects. *Crit. Care Med.,* 2006 34, 403–408.

[56] Morelli, A; Donati, A; Ertmer, C; Rehberg, S; Lange, M; Orecchioni, A; Cecchini, V; Landoni, G; Pelaia, P; Pietropaoli, P; Van Aken, H; Teboul, JL; Ince, C; Westphal, M. Levosimendan for resuscitating the microcirculation in patients with septic shock: a randomized controlled study. *Crit. Care,* 2010 14(6), R232.

[57] Spronk, PE; Ince, C; Gardien, MJ; Mathura, KR; Oudemans-van Straaten, HM; Zandstra, DF. Nitroglycerin in septic shock after intravascular volume resuscitation. *Lancet,* 2002 360, 1395–1396.

[58] Boerma, EC; Koopmans, M; Konijn, A; Kaiferova, K; Bakker, AJ; van Roon, EN; Buter, H; Bruins, N; Egbers, PH; Gerritsen, RT; Koetsier, PM; Kingma, WP; Kuiper, MA; Ince, C. Effects of nitroglycerin on sublingual microcirculatory blood flow in patients with severe sepsis/septic shock after a strict resuscitation protocol: a double-blind randomized placebo controlled trial. *Crit. Care Med.,* 2010 38(1), 93-100.

[59] Comprehensive report on blood collection and transfusion in the US in 2001. Available online at: www.nbdrc.org.

[60] Vincent, JL; Baron, JF; Reinhart, K; Gattinoni, L; Thijs, L; Webb, A; Meier-Hellmann, A; Nollet, G; Peres-Bota, D. Anemia and blood transfusion in critically ill patients. *JAMA,* 2002 288, 1499-1507.

[61] Corwin, HL; Gettinger, A; Pearl, RG; Fink, MP; Levy, MM; Abraham, E; MacIntyre, NR; Shabot, MM; Duh, MS; Shapiro, MJ. The CRIT Study: anemia and blood transfusion in the critically ill – current clinical practice in the United States. *Crit. Care Med.,* 2004 32, 39-52.

[62] Creteur, J; Neves, AP; Vincent, JL. Near-infrared spectroscopy technique to evaluate the effects of red blood cell transfusion on tissue oxygenation. *Critical Care,* 2009 13(Suppl 5), S11.

[63] Sakr, Y; Chierego, M; Piagnerelli, M; Verdant, C; Dubois, MJ; Koch, M; Creteur, J; Gullo, A; Vincent, JL; De Backer, D. Microvascular response to red blood cell transfusion in patients with severe sepsis. *Crit. Care Med.,* 2007 35, 1639-1644.

[64] Sadaka, F; Aggu-Sher, R; Krause, K; O'Brien, J; Armbrecht, ES; Taylor, RW. The effect of red blood cell transfusion on tissue oxygenation and microcirculation in severe septic patients. *Ann. Intensive Care,* 2011 1(1), 46.

[65] Rivers, E; Nguyen, B; Havstadt, S; Ressler, J; Muzzin, A; Knoblich, B; Peterson, E; Tomlanovich, M; Early Goal-Directed Therapy Collaborative Group. Early goal-directed therapy in the treatment of severe sepsis and septic shock. *N. Engl. J. Med.*, 2001 345, 1368–1377.

[66] Hoffmann, JN; Vollmar, B; Laschke, MW; Inthorn, D; Schildberg, FW, Menger, MD. Hydroxyethyl starch (130 kD), but not crystalloid volume support, improves microcirculation during normotensive endotoxemia. *Anesthesiology*, 2002 97, 460–470.

[67] Ospina-Tascon, G; Neves, AP; Occhipinti, G; Donadello, K; Büchele, G; Simion, D; Chierego, ML; Silva, TO; Fonseca, A; Vincent, JL; De Backer, D. Effects of fluids on microvascular perfusion in patients with severe sepsis. *Intensive Care Med.*, 2010 36, 949–955.

[68] Sadaka, F. The Effect of Three Different Fluids (Albumin 5%, Normal Saline, Hydroxyethyl Starch 130 kD) on Microcirculation in Severe Sepsis/Septic Shock Patients. www.clinicaltrials.gov (NCT01319630).

[69] Sprung, CL; Annane, D; Keh, D; Moreno, R; Singer, M; Freivogel, K; Weiss, YG; Benbenishty, J; Kalenka, A; Forst, H; Laterre, PF; Reinhart, K; Cuthbertson, BH; Payen, D; Briegel, J; CORTICUS Study Group. Hydrocortisone therapy for patients with septic shock. *N. Engl. J. Med.*, 2008 358, 111–124.

[70] Büchele, GL; Silva, E; Ospina-Tascón, GA; Vincent, JL; De Backer, D. Effects of hydrocortisone on microcirculatory alterations in patients with septic shock. *Crit. Care Med.*, 2009 37(4), 1341-7.

[71] Lamblin, V; Favory, R; Boulo, M; Mathieu, D. Microcirculatory alterations induced by sedation in intensive care patients. Effects of midazolam alone and in association with sufentanil. *Crit. Care*, 2006 10(6), R176.

[72] Koch, M; De Backer, D; Vincent, JL; Barvais, L; Hennart, D; Schmartz, D. Effects of propofol on human microcirculation. *Br. J. Anaesth*, 2008 101(4), 473-8.

[73] Jung, C; Rödiger, C; Lauten, A; Fritzenwanger, M; Goebel, B; Schumm, J; Figulla, HR; Ferrari, M. Long-term therapy with propofol has no impact on microcirculation in medical intensive care patients. *Med. Klin. (Munic)*, 2009 104(5), 336-42.

[74] Fink, MP. Cytopathic hypoxia in sepsis. *Acta Anaesthesiol Scand Suppl*, 1997 110, 87-95.

[75] Ince, C. Microcirculatory weak units: an alternative explanation. *Crit. Care Med.,* 2000 28, 3128-3129.

[76] Spronk, PE; Kanoore-Edul, VS; Ince, C. Microcirculatory and mitochondrial distress syndrome (MMDS): a new look at sepsis. In *Functional Hemodynamic Monitoring.* Edited by Pinsky MR, Payen D. Berlin: Springer-Verlag; 2004. Update in *Intensive Care Emergency Medicine,* 2004 42, 47-69.

In: Septic Shock
Editors: M. Johnston and J. Knight
ISBN: 978-1-62257-485-8
© 2012 Nova Science Publishers, Inc.

Chapter 6

THE ROLE OF HMGB1 IN CARDIAC DYSFUNCTION DURING SEPTIC SHOCK

Satoshi Hagiwara[*], Hideo Iwasaka and Takayuki Noguchi

Department of Anesthesiology and Intensive Care Medicine,
Oita University Faculty of Medicine, Idaigaoka-Hasamamachi,
Yufu City, Oita, Japan

ABSTRACT

Sepsis, defined as infection complicated by acute organ dysfunction, is a major cause of morbidity and mortality in intensive care patients. Physiologically, sepsis is an acute inflammatory response against an infectious organism accompanied by a complex cascade of cellular and biochemical interactions. Recent studies have demonstrated that the inflammatory response can be accompanied by cardiac dysfunction during septic shock. In particular, myocardial dysfunction frequently occurs in severe sepsis. The extent of cardiac dysfunction varies widely, from isolated and mild diastolic dysfunction to combined severe diastolic and systolic failure of both ventricles. In some cases, it can mimic cardiogenic shock.

---

[*] Corresponding Author: Satoshi Hagiwara; Department of Anesthesiology and Intensive Care Medicine, Oita University Faculty of Medicine, 1-1 Idaigaoka-Hasamamachi, Yufu City, Oita 879-5593 Japan. E-mail address: saku@oita-u.ac.jp; Tel: +81-97-586-5943; Fax: +81-97-586-5949.

High-mobility group protein B1 (HMGB1) is constitutively expressed in many cell types, and localizes to the nucleus via two lysine-rich nuclear localization sequences. HMGB1 binds to chromosomal DNA to regulate nucleosome structure and stability and to control gene expression. However, HMGB1 is also secreted by various cell types during septic shock to mediate lethal sepsis. Here, we review emerging evidence that supports extracellular HMGB1 as a late mediator of experimental sepsis, and discuss cardiac dysfunction during sepsis.

INTRODUCTION

Cardiac dysfunction commonly occurs in the intensive care unit, primarily due to sepsis and septic shock-related organ dysfunction. Sepsis and septic shock are disorders of the innate immune system. Organ dysfunction during sepsis is a life-threatening and extremely costly clinical problem affecting approximately 600,000 patients annually in the United States, with an associated mortality rate estimated at 20% to 60%. Despite the development of many new therapeutic tools over the last 20 years, including initial resuscitation, antibiotic therapy, vasopressors, inotropic therapy, steroids, glucose control, and recombinant human activated protein C, sepsis remains the leading cause of death in intensive care units [1-3]. Recently, therapeutic strategies have been developed to treat sepsis-related cardiac dysfunction.

MECHANISM OF SEPSIS-RELATED CARDIAC DYSFUNCTION

Sepsis is defined as systemic inflammation caused by severe infection. In general, the normal host response to infection is to identify and control pathogen invasion, followed by immediate tissue repair. When both cellular and humoral immune systems are activated, levels of anti-inflammatory and proinflammatory mediators rise in the serum and organs. However, during sepsis and septic shock, the cellular and humoral immune systems are overactivated, causing a massive release of inflammatory mediators, which can lead to multiple organ dysfunctions [4].

Numerous studies have investigated the mechanism of cardiac dysfunction. Damage to cardiomyocytes cannot be explained solely by hypoperfusion related to low systemic vascular resistance. During septic shock, high concentrations of proinflammatory cytokines (e.g., tumor necrosis factor [TNF]-α and interleukin [IL]-1β), impair myocyte contraction and relaxation [5, 6].

Both anti-inflammatory and proinflammatory mediators are activated by intracellular signaling pathways such as the cAMP-dependent kinase, protein kinase A, IκB kinase, protein kinase C, and mitogen-activated protein kinases; the roles of these pathways in regulating myocardial function have also been examined [7-9]. Anticytokine treatment against TNF-α and IL-1β was evaluated, but it did not improve outcomes of patients with sepsis; further, this treatment was shown to disturb cardiomyocyte function [10-13]. Therefore, new therapeutic targets are sought for the treatment of sepsis and sepsis-related organ dysfunction.

THE ROLE OF HMGB1 IN SEPSIS AND AS A POTENTIAL THERAPEUTIC TARGET

High-mobility group protein B1 (HMGB1) is a member of the high mobility group (HMG) discovered more than 35 years ago. HMG proteins are non-histone, chromatin-associated proteins that are constitutively expressed in the nucleus of eukaryotic cells, where they are involved in DNA organization and transcriptional regulation [14]. HMGB1 is implicated in diverse cellular functions, such as regulating nucleosome structure and stability, and facilitating the binding of transcription factors to their cognate DNA sequences [15-17]. The binding of HMGB1 to DNA is regulated by two positively charged domains known as HMG boxes (A box and B box), each of which consists of three α-helices in a characteristic L-shaped fold [18].

In 1999, Wang H et al. first reported that HMGB1 was involved in the pathogenesis of sepsis and septic shock. In contrast to the roles of well-known mediators TNF-α and IL-6, HMGB1 is expressed in the late phase of sepsis and septic shock. In vitro, HMGB1 is secreted by macrophages 20 hours after activation with endotoxin. In vivo, HMGB1 is detected in serum 20 to 72 hours after the onset of the infection, starting just before the onset of lethality from endotoxemia or sepsis. For this reason, HMGB1 is known as a late-phase mediator or lethal mediator [19, 20].

Recent studies have demonstrated that HMGB1 exerts a pro-inflammatory effect [21] and induces neutrophil infiltration and acute injury [22]. Circulating HMGB1 reaches organs and impairs organ function (Figure 1).

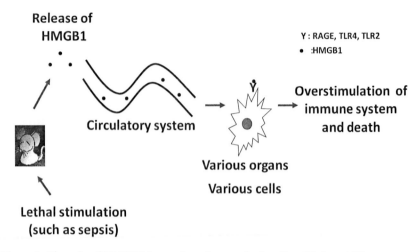

Figure 1. The role of HMGB1 in sepsis and organ dysfunction. High mobility group box 1: HMGB1, Toll-like receptor 4: TLR4, Toll-like receptor 2: TLR2, Receptor for AGE: RAGE.

In particular, HMGB1 produces a negative inotropic effect on cardiomyocytes [23, 24], indicating an important role for this molecule in cardiovascular system dysfunction during sepsis.

On the basis of these findings, HMGB1 has become an important therapeutic target for sepsis and septic shock. Besides improving septic shock, anti-HMGB1 therapy may improve sepsis-related cardiac dysfunction. The anti-HMGB1 agents intravenous immunoglobulin, anti-thrombin III, thrombomodulin, and danaparoid sodium have been shown to reduce serum HMGB1 levels during sepsis and systemic inflammation [25-28]. However, these therapies did not produce beneficial effects in clinical trials. Therefore, further research is needed to develop new anti-HMGB1 agents.

CONCLUSION

Although the mechanism of sepsis is complex and difficult to understand, a recent study indicated that HMGB1 may be a critical mediator of sepsis and septic shock. HMGB1 is also known to cause cardiac dysfunction during sepsis. For these reasons, HMGB1 may be useful as a therapeutic target for sepsis and septic shock. Results so far have been mixed; thus, further study is needed to evaluate HMGB1-targeted therapies for sepsis.

REFERENCES

[1] Martin, G.S., D.M. Mannino, S. Eaton, M. Moss. The epidemiology of sepsis in the United States from 1979 through 2000. *N. Engl. J. Med.* 2003;348:1546–1554.

[2] Moss, M., G.S. Martin. A global perspective on the epidemiology of sepsis. *Intensive Care Med.* 2004;30:527–529.

[3] Watson, R.S., J.A. Carcillo, W.T. Linde-Zwirble, G. Clermont, J. Lidicker, D.C. Angus. The epidemiology of severe sepsis in children in the United States. *Am. J. Respir. Crit. Care Med.* 2003;167:695–701.

[4] Chandra A, Enkhbaatar P, Nakano Y, Traber LD, Traber DL. Sepsis: emerging role of nitric oxide and selectins. *Clinics.* 2006;61:71–76.

[5] Parrillo JE, Burch C, Shelhamer JH, Parker MM, Natanson C, Schuette W. A circulating myocardial depressant substance in humans with septic shock. Septic shock patients with a reduced ejection fraction have a circulating factor that depresses in vitro myocardial cell performance. *J. Clin. Invest.* 1985;76:1539–53.

[6] Kumar A, Michael P, Brabant D, Parissenti AM, Ramana CV, Xu X, Parrillo JE. Human serum from patients with septic shock activates transcription factors STAT1, IRF1, and NF-kappaB and induces apoptosis in human cardiac myocytes. *J. Biol. Chem.* 2005; 280: 42619–26.

[7] Neumann J. Altered phosphatase activity in heart failure, influence on Ca2+ movement. *Basic Res. Cardiol.* 2002;97 1:I91–5.

[8] Jones WK, Brown M, Ren X, He S, McGuinness M. NF-kappaB as an integrator of diverse signaling pathways: the heart of myocardial signaling? *Cardiovasc. Toxicol.* 2003;3:229–54.

[9] Sulakhe PV, Vo XT. Regulation of phospholamban and troponin-I phosphorylation in the intact rat cardiomyocytes by adrenergic and cholinergic stimuli: roles of cyclic nucleotides, calcium, protein kinases and phosphatases and depolarization. *Mol. Cell Biochem.* 1995;149-150:103–26.

[10] Abraham E, Anzueto A, Gutierrez G, et al. Double-blind randomised controlled trial of monoclonal antibody to human tumour necrosis factor in treatment of septic shock. NORASEPT II Study Group. *Lancet* 1998;351:929-33.

[11] Cohen J, Carlet J. INTERSEPT: an international, multicenter, placebo-controlled trial of monoclonal antibody to human tumor necrosis factor-

alpha in patients with sepsis. International Sepsis Trial Study Group. *Crit. Care Med.* 1996;24:1431-40.
[12] CrossRefMedlineWeb of Science.
[13] Fisher CJ, Dhainaut JF, Opal SM, et al. Recombinant human interleukin 1 receptor antagonist in the treatment of patients with sepsis syndrome. Results from a randomized, double-blind, placebo-controlled trial. Phase III rhIL-1ra Sepsis Syndrome Study Group. *J. Am. Med. Assoc.* 1994; 271: 1836-43.
[14] Opal SM, Fisher CJ, Dhainaut JF, et al. Confirmatory interleukin-1 receptor antagonist trial in severe sepsis: a phase III, randomized, double-blind, placebo-controlled, multicenter trial. The Interleukin-1 Receptor Antagonist Sepsis Investigator Group. *Crit. Care Med.* 1997; 25:1115-24.
[15] Goodwin GH, Sanders C, Johns EW. A new group of chromatin-associated proteins with a high content of acidic and basic amino acids. *Eur. J. Biochem.* 1973;38:14–19.
[16] Locker D, Decoville M, Maurizot JC, Bianchi ME, Leng M. Interaction between cisplatin-modified DNA and the HMG boxes of HMG 1: DNase I footprinting and circular dichroism. *J. Mol. Biol.* 1995; 246: 243–247.
[17] Bianchi ME, Beltrame M, Paonessa G. Specific recognition of cruciform DNA by nuclear protein HMG1. *Science.* 1989;243:1056–1059.
[18] Bustin M. Regulation of DNA-dependent activities by the functional motifs of the high-mobility-group chromosomal proteins1. *Mol. Cell Biol.* 1999;19:5237–5246.
[19] Weir HM, Kraulis PJ, Hill CS, Raine AR, Laue ED, Thomas JO. Structure of the HMG box motif in the B-domain of HMG1. *EMBO J.* 1993;12:1311–1319.
[20] Wang H, Bloom O, Zhang M, Vishnubhakat JM, Ombrellino M, Che J, Frazier A, Yang H, Ivanova S, Borovikova L, Manogue KR, Faist E, Abraham E, Andersson J, Andersson U, Molina PE, Abumrad NN, Sama A, Tracey KJ. HMG-1 as a late mediator of endotoxin lethality in mice. *Science.* 1999;285:248–251.
[21] Yang H, Ochani M, Li J, Qiang X, Tanovic M, Harris HE, Susarla SM, Ulloa L, Wang H, DiRaimo R, Czura CJ, Wang H, Roth J, Warren HS, Fink MP, Fenton MJ, Andersson U, Tracey KJ. Reversing established sepsis with antagonists of endogenous high-mobility group box 1. *Proc. Natl. Acad. Sci. U S A.* 2004;101:296–301.

[22] Agnello D, Wang H, Yang H, Tracey KJ, Ghezzi P. HMGB1, a DNA-binding protein with cytokine activity, induces brain TNF and IL-6 production, and mediates anorexia and taste aversion. *Cytokine*. 2002; 18:231–236.

[23] Rowe SM, Jackson PL, Liu G, Hardison M, Livraghi A, Solomon GM, McQuaid DB, Noerager BD, Gaggar A, Clancy J, O'Neal W, Sorscher EJ, Abraham E, Blalock JE. Potential Role of High Mobility Group Box 1 in Cystic Fibrosis Airway Disease. *Am. J. Respir. Crit. Care Med.* 2008; 178(8):822–31.

[24] Hagiwara S, Iwasaka H, Uchino T, Noguchi T.High mobility group box 1 induces a negative inotropic effect on the left ventricle in an isolated rat heart model of septic shock: a pilot study. *Circ J.* 2008 Jun; 72(6): 1012-7.

[25] Tzeng HP, Fan J, Vallejo JG, Dong JW, Chen X, Houser SR, Mann DL.egative inotropic effects of high-mobility group box 1 protein in isolated contracting cardiac myocytes. *Am. J. Physiol. Heart Circ. Physiol.* 2008 Mar; 294(3):H1490-6.

[26] Hagiwara S, Iwasaka H, Hasegawa A, Asai N, Noguchi T. High-dose intravenous immunoglobulin G improves systemic inflammation in a rat model of CLP-induced sepsis. *Intensive Care Med.* 2008;34(10):1812–1819.

[27] Hagiwara S, Iwasaka H, Matsumoto S, Noguchi T. High dose antithrombin III inhibits HMGB1 and improves endotoxin-induced acute lung injury in rats. *Intensive Care Med.* 2008;34:361–367.

[28] Hagiwara S, Iwasaka H, Hasegawa A, Koga H, Noguchi T. Effects of hyperglycemia and insulin therapy on high mobility group box 1 in endotoxin-induced acute lung injury in a rat model. *Crit. Care Med.* 2008; 36:2407–2413.

[29] Hagiwara S, Iwasaka H, Hidaka S, Hishiyama S, Noguchi T.Danaparoid sodium inhibits systemic inflammation and prevents endotoxin-induced acute lung injury in rats.*Crit. Care.* 2008;12(2):R43.

In: Septic Shock
Editors: M. Johnston and J. Knight

ISBN: 978-1-62257-485-8
© 2012 Nova Science Publishers, Inc.

Chapter 7

PATHOPHYSIOLOGY OF SEPSIS AND SEPTIC SHOCK

Jazmina Bongain
Staff member of the Pediatric Intensive Care Unit,
Doctor Roberto del Río Children's Hospital, Santiago de Chile.
Pediatrics and Intensive Care, University of Chile, Chile

ABSTRACT

Sepsis has been recognized as an important public health problem and represents a major factor in morbidity and mortality in intensive care units worldwide in any age group. Recently, the American College of Chest Physicians and the Society of Critical Care Medicine (ACCP/SCCM) reaffirmed the criteria for diagnosing sepsis in order to improve patient care, allow the enrollment in clinical trials and improve communication between ICUs. In this consensus SIRS coined the term to refer to a process inflammatory independent of cause while the term sepsis represents the systemic inflammatory response to the presence of infection.

The host response to sepsis involves many concomitant, integrated, and often antagonistic processes that result both in exaggerated inflammation and immune suppression. The pathogenesis of this condition is now becoming better understood, allowing a greater understanding of the complex network of immune, inflammatory and hematological mediators, which may permit the development of rational and novel therapies. This chapter reviews the pathophysiology of the inflammatory process involved in sepsis and septic shock, laying the groundwork for better understanding of the origin in the generation of free radicals and oxidative stress.

ABBREVIATIONS

ATP	adenosine triphosphate
CARS	compensatory anti-inflammatory response syndrome
C5aR	C5a receptor
EF	ejection fraction
H_2O_2	oxygen peroxide
NFkB	nuclear factor kB
iNOS	inducible nitric oxide synthase isoform
LPS	lipopolysaccharide
MODS	multiple organ dysfunction syndrome
MHC	class II major histocompatibility complex
NO•	nitric oxide
NOS	nitric oxide synthase
O_2•−	superoxide
ONOO−	peroxynitrite
RNS	reactive nitrogen species
ROS	reactive oxygen species
SIRS	systemic inflammatory response syndrome
SOD	superoxide dismutase
TNF	tumor necrosis factor

2. INTRODUCTION

Sepsis has been recognized as an important public health problem and represents a major factor in morbidity and mortality in intensive care units worldwide at any age group. In the United Stated septic shock in adult patients causes more than 200,000 deaths and more than 750.000 sepses every year, with mortality rates as high as 40–60%.[1]. Despite prompt treatment with antibiotics, provision of adequate fluid resuscitation, and technological support of organ function, the mortality rate remains unacceptably high. In children it is also a major cause of mortality up to 80% in some developing countries [2]. In developed countries infant mortality due to sepsis has fallen significantly in recent years [3], but still remains one of the leading causes of morbidity and mortality being around 7% of all death [4].

Annually in the United States, there are 42,000 cases of pediatric severe sepsis, with a reported case fatality rate of 10.3% [4]. In the UK, infection accounts for more than 10% of deaths in children less than 4 years old [5] and approximately 1000 children with severe sepsis are admitted to pediatric intensive care units annually. In 1991, a consensus conference organized by the American College of Chest Physicians and Society of Critical Care Medicine (ACCP/SCCM) reaffirmed the criteria for diagnosing sepsis. It put forward a new syndrome, which was named the 'systemic inflammatory response syndrome' (SIRS) [6]. The concept of SIRS was coined to describe an inflammatory process, triggered by many factors including infections, trauma, surgery and others causing stress. Even though the definition has high sensitivity and low specificity, it has been helpful in improving patient care, allowing enrollment in clinical trials and improving communication between ICUs. Thus the term sepsis represents the systemic inflammatory response in relation to the presence of infection [7]. The clinical manifestations are the result of changes in pathophysiology at the capillary endothelial level and are characterized by the presence of fever, tachycardia, tachypnea and altered leukocyte counts with high suspicion of evidence of a presumed or known site of infection. Patients with sepsis and evidence of organ dysfunction such as respiratory or renal failure are considered to have severe sepsis.

Patients with severe sepsis, who additionally are on persistent hypotension refractory to fluid resuscitation, are in septic shock [7]. Progression of this continuum from sepsis to severe sepsis and septic shock is associated with increased morbidity and mortality. The pathogenesis of this condition, now better known, has allowed an improved understanding of the complex network of immune, inflammatory and hematological mediators that may allow the development of rational and novel therapies. Notwithstanding the foregoing, the mortality has remained high so that early recognition is still the best tool to decrease mortality and length of stay associated with multiple organ failure.

3. PATHOPHYSIOLOGY OF SEPSIS

The normal host response to infection is to both identify and control pathogen invasion and to start immediate tissue repair when necessary. The host response to sepsis involves many concomitant, integrated, and often antagonistic processes that result both in exaggerated inflammation and immune suppression. These defense mechanisms include the release of cytokines, the activation of neutrophils, monocytes, and microvascular endothelial cells, as well as the activation of neuroendocrine reflexes and plasma protein cascade systems, such as the complement system, the intrinsic (contact system) and extrinsic pathways of coagulation, and the fibrinolytic system.

The host response, rather than the nature of the pathogen, primarily determines the patient's outcome. Now it has been recognized that alterations to the patient's immune system, with an excessive systemic inflammatory response on one hand, and paralysis of cell mediated immunity on the other, appear to be the key elements in the pathogenesis of multiple organ failure, susceptibility to infection and associated mortality.

In sepsis, the inflammatory process becomes amplified leading in a continuum from a lowgrade systemic response associated with a self-limited infection to a marked systemic response, representing a spectrum of clinical and pathophysiologic severity. The intensity of the inflammatory response is determined by various host factors (e.g. comorbid diseases, nutritional status and genetics) as well as inciting infection related factors including virulence and bacterial load. [8]

The intense and sustained inflammatory response can result in tissue damage and organ failure. Several factors are implicated in the pathogenesis of organ failure, such as the endocrine and immune systems, disseminated intravascular coagulation, genetic susceptibility and mitochondrial dysfunction and an acquired transient intrinsic defect in cellular respiration termed "cytopathic hypoxia" [9].

Following acute sepsis, a 'compensatory anti-inflammatory response syndrome' (CARS) develops, leading to immunosuppression [10]. This is an adaptive mechanism whose purpose is to regulate and protect against inflammatory injury, but with risk of newly acquired nosocomial infections and mortality in sepsis.

3.1. Basic Molecular Mechanisms of Inflammation in Sepsis

The innate immune system is the primordial and the first line of defense against invading pathogens [11]. Its function is thought to be the recognition of invading pathogens, the activation of inflammation to control the pathogen, and the subsequent activation of the acquired immune response. It includes cell types playing primary roles in phagocytosis and intracellular killing (polymorphonuclear cells), cytotoxic killing (natural killer cells), and antigen presentation (dendritic) cells [12].

The monocytes and their descendants play a key role in the activation and initiation of the innate immune response. Its function includes the recognition and phagocytosis of pathogens, secretion of mediators that modulate the overall immune response and presentation of digested peptides on its cell surface to activate the adaptive immune response.

Once stimulated, monocytes engulf and destroy microbes, which then are processed into antigenic peptides. These are presented on the external surfaces of innate immune cells in conjunction with class II major histocompatibility complex molecules, such as HLA-DR. Antigens presented in this way, along with co-stimulatory input from the innate immune cells, activate the adaptive arm of the immune response [12].

3.1.1. Pathogen-Host Interaction

The recognition of microbial products by the innate arm of the immune system is an essential element for the setting of the host defense. After recognizing the pathogen, it occurs the production of cytokines and chemokines involved in the leukocyte promotion and recruitment to the infection focus, thus inducing their microbicidal activity.

The innate immune response begins with the recognition of the cellular constituents of the pathogen. This is accomplished through the presence of constitutively expressed receptors present on the plasma membranes of innate immune effectors cells. These receptors recognize broad classes of microbial constituents. These microbial components are known as pathogen-associated molecular patterns (PAMPs) and are key elements and constant in the structure of microorganisms [13].

These PAMPs are recognized by pattern recognition receptors (PRRs). These receptors also recognize eukaryotic cell key constituents released as a result of tissue damage and apoptosis. Such endogenous danger signals have been termed "alarmins" or danger-associated molecular patterns (DAMPs) [14]. Several families of PRRs, including Toll-like receptors and cytoplasm receptors, recognize distinct microbial components and directly activate immune cells [15]. This is accomplished through the presence of constitutively expressed receptors present on the plasma membranes of innate immune effector cells. These receptors mediated by phagocytes including macrophages and dendritic cells, initiate the innate immune response and regulate the adaptive immune response to infection. The TLR is the most important molecular mechanism by which the host recognizes the presence of a pathogenic organism and initiates the innate immune response. To date, almost 13 mammalian TLRs have been identified, and each is known to detect a specific intracellular signaling pathway. Toll-Like receptor 1,2,4,5 and 6 mainly recognize bacterial product, whereas TLR- 3, TLR-7 and TLR-8 are specific for viral detection. Toll like receptor 9 seems to be involved in both microbial and viral recognition, while TLR4 is the most important sensor of Gram-negative bacterial products [16], whereas TLR2 seems to be the key receptor in activating the immune system against Gram-positive bacteria [17]. TLR 4 may further contribute to the pathogenesis of sepsis by amplifying inflammatory responses through interaction with DAMPs released after tissue injury [18] besides acting as sensor of oxidative stress [19]. Binding of TLRs activates intracellular signal-transduction pathways that lead to the activation of cytosolic nuclear factor-kb (NF-κb). Activated NF-κb moves from the cytoplasm to the nucleus, binds to transcription sites and induces activation of hundreds of genes that are important in immune inflammatory responses [20]. These include genes for cytokines, adhesion molecules and chemokines, receptors required for neutrophil adhesion and transmigration across blood vessel walls, receptors involved in immune recognition, such as members of the major histocompatibility complex; and proteins involved in antigen presentation [21]. NF-κB also modulates antimicrobial and immunologic functions by controlling the survival of neutrophils and the proliferation and differentiation of B- and T-lymphocytes at the site of the infection [22].

3.1.2. Neutrophils

The neutrophil is an integral component of the innate immune system, the first and most abundant leukocyte to be delivered to a site of infection or inflammation [23].

These cells have a pivotal role in the defense against bacterial infections, as shown by neutropenia (eg, after chemotherapy), which increases the susceptibility to local infection and to sepsis. Bacterial elimination is dependent on the rapid recruitment of blood neutrophils into sites of infection. During inflammation, circulating bloodstream neutrophils contact and transiently interact with endothelial cell molecules resulting in a cell rolling on the blood vessel wall. This initial cell contact represents the first step in a cascade of molecular interactions leading to leukocyte extravasations, and is a critical prerequisite for a tighter interaction. Circulating neutrophils are attracted to the site of inflammation in response to chemoattractant mediators locally released such as the complement peptide C5a, leukotriene B4, platelet-activating factor, the bacterial peptide formyl-methionyl-leucyl-phenylalanine, and interleukin 8 [24]. The cells migrate from an area of low concentration (ie, blood vessel walls) to an area of high concentration (site of infection or inflammation), whereupon the chemotactic factors become potent neutrophil activators [25]. Once activated, neutrophils are able to phagocytose, release granular lytic enzymes and antimicrobial polypeptides into the phagolysosome, and to generate large amounts of reactive oxygen and nitrogen species, such as hydrogen peroxide (H_2O_2) and nitric oxide (NO), which are crucial products for the microbicidal activity of these cells.

Neutrophil priming causes an increase in the response of these cells to an activating agent and prolongs their lifespan by inhibiting apoptosis, as well as inducing an up-regulation in their expression of vascular adhesion molecules: the selectins and integrins [12]. Both families of adhesion molecules control the binding of neutrophils to the vascular endothelium. The selectins promote the initial rolling or tethering of the neutrophils to the endothelium under the shear force of blood flow, whereas the integrins induce firm adhesion [26].

Neutrophils are ideally suited to the elimination of pathogenic bacteria for their large stores of proteolytic enzymes and rapid production of reactive oxygen species to degrade internalyzed pathogens. If these lytic factor or pro-inflammatory cytokines are released in the tissue infiltrating neutrophils, local damage will ensue. By contrast, in severe sepsis local infection is accompanied by systemic neutrophil activation.

The overwhelming activation of neutrophils is known to elicit tissue damage. Clinical evidence related aberrant neutrophil activity with the organ failure of severe sepsis [27].

Removal of neutrophils by apoptosis is a homoeostatic mechanism preventing damage to healthy tissues that would otherwise occur after the lysis of necrotic cells. This process is central for the prevention and resolution of inflammation. Neutrophil apoptosis is inhibited in patients with systemic inflammation, systemic infections, severe sepsis, and those at risk of multiple organ failure [28].

3.1.3. Cytokines

Cytokines and chemokines are important components of the immune system that act as messages between cells, both in the innate and adaptive immune systems. So these molecules are the extracellular expression of the immune system.

The early phase of sepsis is dominated by a hyper-inflammatory state mediated by the systemic production of inflammatory cytokines. Interleukin 1 (IL-1), IL-6, tumor necrosis factor alpha (TNF-α), and gamma interferon (IFN-γ) have pro-inflammatory effects.

These cytokines and chemokines modulate the inflammatory response by recruiting and activating other immune effectors cells and activating non cellular aspects of the immune response, such as the complement and coagulation cascades [12, 29]. The most important pro-inflammatory cytokines are TNF and IL-1.

These cytokines have many local actions, including stimulation of synthesis of other cytokines, up-regulation of the expression of tissue factor and adhesion molecules on nearby cells, induction of certain enzymes (eg, phospholipase A2, cycloxygenase-2). TNF-α and other pro-inflammatory molecules can also activate downstream effectors of acute inflammation, for example, by up-regulating the expression of inducible nitric oxide synthase, which results in an increased release of NO and its attendant effects on the micro-vascular resistance and capillary flow, or by augmenting neutrophil cytotoxic mechanisms by inducing the release of oxygen radicals and proteolytic enzymes [29, 30].

TNF-α results in activation of nearby immune cells and pro-inflammatory changes in the vascular endothelium promoting cellular migration into the periphery. When this modulation becomes a systemic one, the clinical signs and symptoms of hyper-inflammation (fever, hemodynamic instability, capillary leak between others) become evident [12]. Concomitant with the initial hyper-inflammatory response, there is a nearly simultaneous production of anti-inflammatory cytokines, including IL-10, that serve to balance the inflammatory state.

Both, the inflammatory and anti-inflammatory phase, are coordinated to defend the host against invasion by pathogens. However, an excessive or sustained inflammatory response, an inadequate anti-inflammatory response, or perhaps an uncoupling of these 2 phases may contribute to tissue damage and cell death [29].

3.1.4. Coagulation Disorders in Sepsis

The coagulopathy in critical illness is biologically complex. Besides activating the inflammatory system, pathogens also trigger early activation of the contact system (factor XII, prekallikrein, and high-molecular-weight kininogen) and the complement cascade [31]. Blood coagulation is initiated by activation of the extrinsic pathway and is amplified through the intrinsic pathway. Activation of the extrinsic pathway is initiated through tissue factor expressed on the surface of endothelial cells and monocytes, a process that can be induced by microbial products such as endotoxin, inflammatory cytokines or by integrin crosslinking [32].

The shift toward a procoagulant state results in excessive thrombin generation, fibrin formation, and consumption of clotting factors. Fibrin deposits isolate the source of infection in an attempt to prevent its spread. The disseminated intravascular coagulation in critically ill patients impedes an adequate oxygen delivery to tissues and can induce further inflammatory injury. Within the mechanisms involved in the amplification of the inflammatory response is hypoxia, as a factor indirectly related while the thrombin receptor activation and clustering of tissue factor directly stimulate the expression of multiple pro-inflammatory cytokine genes through the activation of nuclear transcription factor NFκB [33].

3.1.5. Endothelial Cells

Endothelial cells are the predominant lining cells in close and intimate contact with blood. Under normal conditions, the endothelium is highly active serving a variety of functions: among others it mediates vasomotor tone, regulates cellular and nutrient trafficking, maintains blood fluidity, contributes to the local balance of pro-inflammatory and anti-inflammatory mediators, participates in the generation of new blood vessels, and undergoes programmed cell death [34].

In recent years, it has been recognized that endothelial cells produce important regulators of both coagulation and inflammation, thus playing a key role in the pathophysiology of sepsis.

In fact, such a dysfunction could explain most of the clinical manifestations and complications of sepsis. In pro-inflammatory states the endothelial cells undergo functional changes. These changes occur after making contact with cytokines and other pro-inflammatory mediators and are known as endothelial activation. The activated endothelium produces an array of inflammatory mediators. Clearly, the endothelium should not be thought of as an inactive cell layer constituting the vessel wall but rather as a director orchestrating the inflammatory cascade. The physiologic goal of these changes, which are meant to occur locally and not systemically, is to wall off an infectious process.

There is evidence of significant microcirculatory disorders in the course of septic shock. A decrease of the density of perfused capillaries with sluggish or stop-flow perfusion patterns has been observed in septic patients [35]. The microvasculature responds to inflammatory stimuli mainly through activation of the endothelium. On the front line is the expression of adhesion molecules which will enhance endothelial–leukocyte interaction. P-selectin and E-selectin, intercellular adhesion molecule-1, or vascular cellular adhesion molecule-1 are up-regulated by gene-transcription under regulation of transcription factors such as NF-κβ [36]. Interaction of the endothelial adhesion molecules E-selectin with its ligand ESL-1 on leukocytes initiated a second phase of activation after it upregulated the alpha M beta2 integrin on neutrophils, allowing the interaction with RBCs and platelets. These interactions will in turn induce the production of ROS by neutrophils and lead to impairment of the capillary blood flow and vascular damage [37].

Other NF-κβ-regulated genes in endothelial cells include plasminogen activator inhibitor-1, cyclooxygenase-2, and inducible nitric oxide synthase, all involved in the microcirculatory blood flow regulation [36].

Among the factors involved in the alteration of the microcirculation are recognized red blood cells and platelets aggregation, endothelial cell swelling, arteriole vasoconstriction, injury of the endothelium, and increased microvascular permeability with interstitial edema [38]. Activation of the coagulation cascade is another hallmark of sepsis with the inflammatory response activating tissue factor on endothelial cells and monocytes, intravascular thrombin generation, depletion of anticoagulant factors, and alterations of the fibrinolytic system [39].

Alteration of the flow at the microcirculation causes initially a mismatch between cell oxygen demand and supply [40]. Tissue hypoxia stimulates the inflammatory pathways exacerbating the inflammatory state characteristic of this pathology.

Upon stimulation with cytokines such as TNF-α or IL-1, endothelial cells may produce another type of NO-synthase: the inducible NO-synthase. It's expression likely explains the drop in blood pressure in sepsis [41]. Despite large amount of NO produced by inducible nitric oxide synthase during sepsis, generation of superoxide by adhesive leukocytes can decrease endothelium-derived NO bioavailability and compromise microcirculatory blood flow by inducing vasoconstriction or loose of vasodilatation [42].

Several mechanisms may contribute to endothelial damage during sepsis. *In vitro* experiments have shown that activated neutrophils that adhere to the endothelial cells via adhesion molecules are well able to injure the endothelial cells by producing oxygen radicals and proteinases such as elastase [43].

Another mechanism that may cause severe damage to the endothelium is apoptosis induced by TNF-α [44]. Cytokine-activated natural killer cells or cytotoxic T lymphocytes, together known as lymphokines, can adhere to and injure the endothelium, resulting, for example, in increased permeability [45].

3.1.6. Complement Activation

Complement is a complex series of self-assembling plasma proteins which play a major role in host defense against infection and in inflammation.

All three pathways of complement activation (classical, lectin and alternative) converge to generate the C3 convertase and C5 convertase, resulting in biologically active split products of C3 and C5. The major purpose of the complement pathway is to remove or destroy antigen by direct cell killing (complement-mediated lysis), opsonization and complement-dependent phagocytosis, elicitation of an inflammatory response (smooth muscle spasm, release of vasoactive amines, increase of vascular permeability, stimulation of neutrophils and macrophages, etc.), and stimulation of the immune response (such as antigen presentation, T-cell activation, B-cell activation, antibody responses and immunologic memory) [46].

C3b is known to be a vital opsonic product that coats bacteria and other microbes, resulting in uptake by phagocytic cells (neutrophils and macrophages), followed by oxygen-dependent intracellular killing of bacteria [47]. The C5a fragment of the complement is implicated as a particularly potent mediator of the inflammatory process, reacting with high affinity receptors on phagocytic cells, resulting in cell activation which causes generation of reactive oxygen species ($O_2\bullet$, H_2O_2, $HO\bullet$) that are toxic to other cells, enzyme secretion from phagocytic cells, which results in tissue damage. C5a is highly chemotactic for phagocytic cells, especially neutrophils. Collectively, the outcome of C5a generation in vivo is induction of the acute inflammatory response characterized by increased vascular permeability and accumulation and activation of neutrophils and tissue macrophages [48].

3.2. Immunoparalysis

Almost concurrently with the initial hyper-inflammatory response, compensatory mechanisms play a role and shut down the immune system inflammatory response, often through the induction of anti-inflammatory cytokines. This phenomenon is referred to as the "compensatory anti-inflammatory response syndrome" (CARS) [12]. This period of transient immune suppression helps to counterbalance the inflammatory state avoiding a significant end-organ damage and death in a subset of patients [29].

The immunoparalysis represents a persistently severe form of CARS, which is associated with an increased frequency of nosocomial infections and mortality in sepsis. The immunoparalysis is characterized by a marked deterioration in the innate immune function, now recognized as a predictor of morbidity and mortality for children and adults [49, 50]. Clinical research in adults and children with septic shock and MODS have shown that survivors retain the ability to assemble and maintain an innate immune response, with expression of proinflammatory genes [51, 52].

The underlying mechanisms of immunoparalysis are poorly understood. Possible mechanisms responsible include inhibition of the proinflammatory transcription factor NFkB, through alteration of its subunit composition [53], up-regulation of its inhibitor IκBa [54], up-regulation of the NFκB pathway inhibitor IRAK-M, or impairment of TLR4 signaling [55].

This dysfunction is related to a reduction in the monocyte antigen presenting capacity, internalization of cell-surface HLA-DR molecules in normal human monocytes with co-incubation with serum from septic patients [50]. Fumeaux and colleagues [56] demonstrated internalization of cell-surface HLA-DR molecules in normal human monocytes with co-incubation with serum from septic patients. On the other hand, steroids may also play a role in the development or perpetuation of immunoparalysis. Le Tulzo et al [57] found an association between high levels of circulating cortisol and a reduction in monocyte HLA-DR expression in 48 septic patients on day 6 of illness. Others have shown that the administration of methylprednisolone in the setting of a cardiopulmonary bypass procedure resulted in an exacerbation of innate immunosuppression higher than that seen with a bypass alone [58].

In critically ill adults and children lymphocyte apoptosis and lymphopenia are common in ICU non-survivors. Programmed cell death (apoptosis) is a prominent feature in human and experimental sepsis, especially as it involves the lymphoid system with resulting immunoparalysis. In addition, sepsis is associated with strong activation of the complement system, resulting in the generation of the powerful anaphylatoxin, C5a, as well as the up-regulation of the C5a receptor (C5aR) in a variety of different organs.

The consequences of C5a interactions with C5aR can be directly linked to apoptosis of thymocytes and adrenal medullary cells in an experimental model after cecal ligation and puncture-induced sepsis in rodents, resulting in signaling paralysis of blood neutrophils and loss of their innate immune functions (phagocytosis, chemotaxis, respiratory burst), together with apoptosis of thymocytes [48, 59]. The temporal and causal relationship between the innate and adaptive immune dysfunction in critical illness remains incompletely understood.

During the past few decades several assays related to the measurement of immune responsiveness have been reported. Volk and colleagues have defined immunoparalysis in adults as prolonged monocyte HLA-DR expression below 30%, or reduction in whole blood ex vivo LPS-induced TNF-α response to 200 pg/mL for more than 5 days [60], while Hall and cols recently presented similar findings in children who present with a variety of secondary MODS [61].

4. PATHOPHYSIOLOGY OF SEPTIC SHOCK

Septic shock is defined in adults as hypotension refractory to fluid resuscitation. In initial phases in children this may be absent. Its evolution is characterized by progressive hemodynamic and cardiovascular instability. At an early stage clinical signs include tachicardia, full bounding pulses, flushed skin, irritability or drowsiness, narrowed differential blood pressure and in a later stage hypotension, oliguria, clammy skin, low volume pulses, and the patients overall appear to be unstable in their basic condition.

During the initial stages of septic shock, reflex neurohumoral responses occur, that attempt to sustain perfusion by maintaining cardiac output and blood pressure. Activation of baroreceptor reflexes, release of catecholamines, activation of renin-angiotensin, release of antidiuretic hormone, and generalized sympathetic stimulation are included.

Two fundamental pathogenic processes contribute to the clinical manifestations of septic shock: cardiovascular dysfunction due to the combined effects of myocardial depression and systemic vasodilatation and inflammatory tissue damage. The concept of depressed myocardial function in sepsis emerged from studies performed with radionuclide ventriculograms in septic shock patients. Human septic myocardial depression is characterized by reversible biventricular dilatation, increased end diastolic volume, decreased ejection fraction, and decreased response to fluid resuscitation and catecholamine stimulation, despite a normal total cardiac output while compensated [62, 63].

Initial impaired left ventricular systolic and diastolic dysfunction may also be observed with similar alterations in right ventricular function. Different studies have shown that the decrease in EF is reversible with full functional recovery of cardiac function in survivors at 7–10 days after the episode. The presence of a cardiovascular dysfunction in adult sepsis is associated with a significantly increased mortality rate to 70% to 90% compared with 20% in septic patients without cardiovascular impairment. This has been corroborated with echocardiographies in other studies [64]. In this context, myocardial dysfunction was once considered as a preterminal event [63].

Cardiac depression during sepsis is probably multifactorial and involves multiple pathways. The first proposed mechanism is that of global ischemia, however studies in animals and humans showed a high coronary blood flow and diminished coronary artery– coronary sinus oxygen difference [65, 66]. Coronary sinus blood studies in patients with septic shock have also demonstrated increased lactate extraction, decreased free fatty acid extraction, and decreased glucose uptake. Furthermore, studies in animal models of sepsis have demonstrated the presence of normal high-energy phosphate levels in the myocardium. The absence of significant myocardial cell death and the reversible nature of myocardial dysfunction in sepsis support a prominent role for functional rather than anatomical abnormalities in the underlying pathophysiology mechanisms [67-69]. It has also been proposed that myocardial dysfunction in sepsis may reflect hibernating myocardium [70]. Furthermore, evidence of widespread myocardial necrosis has not been found in patients with septic shock. There is no evidence supporting global ischemia as an underlying cause of myocardial dysfunction in sepsis. Parrillo et al using rat cardiac myocytes exposed to serum from septic patients achieved correlating clinical severity quantitatively linked the clinical degree of septic myocardial dysfunction with the decrease in extent and velocity of myocyte shortening. These effects were not seen when serum from convalescent patients whose cardiac function had returned to normal was applied or when serum was obtained from other critically ill nonseptic patients [71]. From these studies the concept of circulating myocardial depressant factor was proposed for sepsis which could be responsible for this phenomenon. Subsequent studies identified cytokines such as TNF-α, IL-1b, and IL-6 as circulating causative factors of myocardial depression in sepsis. On the other hand Mink et al [72] demonstrated that lysozyme c, a bacteriolytic agent believed to originate mainly from disintegrating neutrophilic granulocytes and monocytes, mediates cardiodepressive effects during Escherichia coli sepsis. Early studies suggest a potential role for endothelin-1 (ET-1) in the development of sepsis-induced myocardial depression [73].

Among the factors involved in the myocardial depression of sepsis are nitric oxide, mitochondrial dysfunction, calcium, prostanoids such as thromboxane and prostacyclin and apoptosis. The most promising candidate is NO, which is produced in excessive amounts during sepsis as the consequence of induced expression of NOS in the myocardium. Effects of nitric oxide relevant to sepsis-induced myocardial dysfunction include vasodilation, the depression of mitochondrial respiration, and further release of pro-inflammatory cytokines. The NO also exerts its action indirectly through free radical peroxynitrite formed from NO and superoxide [74]. The description of the mechanisms involved in myocardial depression by the action of NO are beyond the scope of this chapter. In chapter 13 (myocardial dysfunction), these mechanisms are described, while in chapter 6 (multiorgan failure) the general mechanisms of mitochondrial dysfunction are described, along with cellular and organic dysfunction associated with inflammation and oxidative stress.

Calcium is thought to play an important role in the development of sepsis-induced myocardial depression. Current evidence suggests reductions in cytosolic calcium levels during sepsis leading to reduced contractility. Calcium signaling and metabolism is linked to mitochondrial function, which is also altered in sepsis.

Elevated levels of prostanoids such as thromboxane and prostacyclin, which have the potential to alter coronary autoregulation, coronary endothelial function, and intracoronary leukocyte activation, have been demonstrated in septic patients [75]. Unfortunately, studies in both septic patients and experimental animals have failed to demonstrate survival improvement.

Early septic shock is characterized by circulatory abnormalities that usually relate to intravascular volume depletion and vasodilation. As mentioned in the previous section of this chapter the normal function of the endothelium is to regulate the microcirculation by dictating the tonus of the arterioles, regulation of blood pressure (via their effects on arterioles), and regulation of vascular permeability. This function is performed through vasoactive compounds that regulate the tonus of the arterioles and hence have a great influence on blood pressure. These compounds include the vasodilating NO and prostacyclin and the vasoconstricting endothelins [76]. Inflammatory mediators strongly stimulate endothelial production of these molecules.

The production of NO can be regulated by two different mechanisms: constitutive NO-synthase, an enzyme that produces NO in a calcium-dependent manner, and inducible NO-synthase activated by the effect of proinflammatory cytokines, such as TNF-α or IL-1.This enzyme produces large quantities of NO in a calcium-independent manner. Expression of inducible NO synthase likely explains the drop in blood pressure in sepsis [77]. It is noticeable also that NO and prostacyclin also are potent inhibitors of platelet aggregation.

Early sepsis and septic shock are characterized by circulatory abnormalities that usually relate to intravascular volume depletion and vasodilation. This causes an oxygen supply-demand imbalance in various organ beds often reversed by fluid resuscitation when on-time. Insufficiently resuscitated animal models are therefore likely to evidence reduced cardiac performance [78].

Thus, in the early phase of shock, adequate volume replacement has proved to be far more effective for a successful resuscitation, than in later stages of shock, when the compensatory mechanisms have been overwhelmed.

Aggressive volume administration as indicated by international guidelines without taking into account the myocardial compromise/depression may precipitate an additional cardiorespiratory dysfunction with pulmonary edema secondary to myocardial failure and a relative fluid overload for their underlying disease.

Maitland et al in a study in critically ill children with impaired perfusion found that patients who received volume of 20 to 40 ml per kg according to guidelines presented significantly increased 48-hour mortality [79].

CONCLUSION AND FUTURE GOALS

Sepsis and septic shock continue to be responsible for a considerable number of deaths in all age groups around the world. This is despite of advances in the comprehension of the underlying pathophysiologic mechanisms due to extensive research in the field. The aim of the research is to modify or stop the pathophysiologic mechanisms involved in the inflammatory and metabolic disorders to prevent the cellular damage responsible for MODS and deaths. Oxidative stress as part of the pathophysiological process, while extensively studied in biological research, has not just reached clinical settings with a successful therapeutic approach. Since the generation of ROS and RNS, and oxidative stress as a consequence of an imbalance of the oxidative –antioxidative response, play an important role in the pathophysiology of many diseases including sepsis and septic shock, enhancing the knowledge of clinicians about this topic and stimulating future research in the field must continue to be a goal.

REFERENCES

[1] Angus DC, Wax RS. Epidemiology of sepsis: an update. Crit. Care Med. 2001; 29:S109-S116.
[2] Khilnani P, Sarma D, Zimmerman J. Epidemiology and peculiarities of pediatric multiple organ dysfunction syndrome in New Delhi, India. *Intensive Care Med.* 2006; 32:1856-1862.
[3] Brierley J, Carcillo JA, Choong K, Cornell T, Decaen A, Deymann A, Doctor A, Davis A, Duff J, Dugas MA, Duncan A, Evans B, Feldman J, Felmet K, Fisher G, Frankel L, Jeffries H, Greenwald B, Gutierrez J, Hall M, Han YY, Hanson J, Hazelzet J, Hernan L, Kiff J, Kissoon N, Kon A, Irazuzta J, Lin J, Lorts A, Mariscalco M, Mehta R, Nadel S, Nguyen T, Nicholson C, Peters M, Okhuysen-Cawley R, Poulton T, Relves M, Rodriguez A, Rozenfeld R, Schnitzler E, Shanley T, Kache S, Skippen P, Torres A, von Dessauer B, Weingarten J, Yeh T, Zaritsky A, Stojadinovic B, Zimmerman J, Zuckerberg A. Clinical practice parameters for hemodynamic support of pediatric and neonatal septic shock: 2007 update from American College of Critical Care Medicine. *Crit. Care Med.* 2009; 37:666-688.
[4] Watson RS, Carcillo JA, Linde-Zwirble WT, Clermont G, Lidicker J, Angus DC. The epidemiology of severe sepsis in children in the United States. *Am. J. Respir. Crit. Care Med.* 2003; 167:695-170.
[5] Bryce J, Boschi-Pinto C, Shibuya K, Black RE, WHO Child Health Epidemiology Reference Group. WHO estimates of the causes of death in children. *Lancet.* 2005; 365:1147-1152.
[6] American college of chest physicians/society of critical care medicine consensus conference: definitions for sepsis and organ failure and guidelines for the use of innovative therapies in sepsis. *Crit. Care Med.* 1992; 20:864-874.
[7] Bone RC, Balk RA, Cerra FB, Dellinger RP, Fein AM, Knaus WA, Schein RM, Sibbald WJ. Definitions for sepsis and organ failure and guidelines for the use of innovative therapies in sepsis. The ACCP/SCCM Consensus Conference Committee. American College of Chest Physicians/Society of Critical Care Medicine. *Chest.* 1992; 101:1644-1655.

[8] van der Poll T, Opal SM. Host-pathogen interactions in sepsis. *Lancet Infect. Dis.* 2008; 8:32-43.
[9] Brown KA, Brain SD, Pearson JD, Edgeworth JD, Lewis SM, Treacher DF. Neutrophils in development of multiple organ failure in sepsis. *Lancet.* 2006; 368:157-169.
[10] Bone RC. Sir Isaac Newton, sepsis, SIRS, and CARS. *Crit. Care Med.* 1996; 24:1125-1128.
[11] Janeway CA Jr, Medzhitov R. *Annu. Rev. Immunol.* 2002; 20:197-216.
[12] Frazier WJ, Hall MW. Immunoparalysis and adverse outcomes from critical illness. *Pediatr. Clin. North Am.* 2008; 55:647-668.
[13] Janeway CA, Medzhitov R. Introduction: The role of innate immunity in the adaptive immune response. *Semin. Immunol.* 1998; 10:349-350.
[14] Bianchi ME. DAMPs, PAMPs and alarmins: all we need to know about danger. *J. Leukoc. Biol.* 2007; 81:1-5.
[15] Akira S, Uematsu S, Takeuchi O. Pathogen recognition and innate immunity. *Cell.* 2006; 124:783-801.
[16] Poltorak A, Ricciardi-Castagnoli P, Citterio S, Beutler B. Physical contact between lipopoly-saccharide and Toll-like receptor 4 revealed by genetic complementation. *Proc. Nat. Acad. Sci. US.* 2000; 97: 2163-2167.
[17] Schwandner R, Dziarski R, Wesche H, Rothe M, Kirschning CJ. Peptidoglycan- and lipoteichoic acid-induced cell activation is mediated by Toll-like receptor 2. *J. Biol. Chem.* 1999; 274:17406-17409.
[18] Mollen KP, Anand RJ, Tsung A, Prince JM, Levy RM, Billiar TR. Emerging paradigm: Toll-like receptor 4-sentinel for the detection of tissue damage. *Shock.* 2006; 26:430-437.
[19] Imai Y, Kuba K, Neely GG, Yaghubian-Malhami R, Perkmann T, van Loo G, Ermolaeva M, Veldhuizen R, Leung YH, Wang H, Liu H, Sun Y, Pasparakis M, Kopf M, Mech C, Bavari S, Peiris JS, Slutsky AS, Akira S, Hultqvist M, Holmdahl R, Nicholls J, Jiang C, Binder CJ, Penninger JM. Identification of oxidative stress and Toll-like receptor 4 signaling as a key pathway of acute lung injury. *Cell.* 2008; 133: 235-249.
[20] Zingarelli B, Sheehan M, Wong HR. Nuclear factor-☐B as a therapeutic target in critical care medicine. *Crit Care Med. 2003*; 31:S105-S111.
[21] Zingarelli B. Nuclear factor-kappaB. *Crit. Care Med.* 2005; 33:414-416.
[22] Caamaño J, Hunter CA. NF-kappaB family of transcription factors: central regulators of innate and adaptive immune functions. *Clin. Microbiol. Rev.* 2002; 15:414-429.

[23] Seely AJ, Pascual JL, Christou NV. Science review: Cell membrane expression (connectivity) regulates neutrophil delivery, function and clearance. *Crit. Care.* 2003; 7:291-307.

[24] Brown KA, Brain SD, Pearson JD, Edgeworth JD, Lewis SM, Treacher DF. Neutrophils in development of multiple organ failure in sepsis. *Lancet.* 2006; 368:157-169.

[25] Bokoch GM. Chemoattractant signaling and leukocyte activation. *Blood.* 1995; 86:1649-1660.

[26] Barreiro O, Sanchez – Madrid F. Signals emanating from leukocyte-endothelium interactions during inflammation. *An. R.Acad. Farm.* 2008; 74:1-16.

[27] Brown KA, Brain SD, Pearson JD, Edgeworth JD, Lewis SM, Treacher DF. Neutrophils in development of multiple organ failure in sepsis. *Lancet.* 2006; 368:157-169.

[28] Martins PS, Kalla EG, Neto MC, Dalboni MA, Blecher S, Salamao R. Upregulation of reactive oxygen species generation and phagocytosis and an increased apoptosis in human neutrophils during severe sepsis and septic shock. *Shock.* 2003; 20:208-212.

[29] Muenzer JT, Davis CG, Chang K, Schmidt RE, Dunne WM, Coopersmith CM, Hotchkiss RS. Characterization and Modulation of the Immunosuppressive Phase of Sepsis. *Infect. Immun.* 2010; 78:1582-1592.

[30] Mallick AA, Ishizaka A, Stephens KE, Hatherill JR, Tazelaar HD, Raffin TA. Multiple organ damage caused by tumor necrosis factor and prevented by prior neutrophil depletion. *Chest.* 1989; 95:1114-1120.

[31] Aird WC. Vascular bed-specific hemostasis: role of endothelium in sepsis pathogenesis. *Crit. Care Med.* 2001; 29:S28-S35.

[32] Esmon CT. Possible involvement of cytokines in diffuse intravascular coagulation and thrombosis. *Baillieres Best Pract Res Clin Haematol.* 2000; 12:343-359.

[33] McGilvray ID, Rotstein OD. Signaling pathways of tissue factor expression in monocytes and macrophages. *Sepsis.* 1999; 3:93-101.

[34] Cines DB, Pollak ES, Buck CA, Loscalzo J, Zimmerman GA, McEver RP, Pober JS, Wick TM, Konkle BA, Schwartz BS, Barnathan ES, McCrae KR, Hug BA, Schmidt AM, Stern DM. Endothelial cells in physiology and in the pathophysiology of vascular disorders. *Blood.* 1998; 91:3527-3561.

[35] Boerma EC, van der Voort PH, Spronk PE, Ince C. Relationship between sublingual and intestinal microcirculatory perfusion in patients with abdominal sepsis. *Crit. Care Med.* 2007; 35:1055-1060.

[36] De Martin R, Hoeth M, Hofer-Warbinek R, Schmid JA. The transcription factor NF-kappa B and the regulation of vascular cell function. *Arterioscler. Thromb. Vasc. Biol.* 2000; 20:E83-E88.

[37] Tyml K, Li F, Wilson JX. Septic impairment of capillary blood flow requires nicotinamide adenine dinucleotide phosphate oxidase but not nitric oxide synthase and is rapidly reversed by ascorbate through an endothelial nitric oxide synthase-dependent mechanism. *Crit. Care Med.* 2008; 36:2355-2362.

[38] Balestra GM, Legrand M, Ince C. Microcirculation and mitochondria in sepsis: getting out of breath. *Curr. Opin. Anaesthesiol.* 2009; 22:184-190.

[39] Opal SM, Garber GE, LaRosa SP, Maki DG, Freebairn RC, Kinasewitz GT, Dhainaut JF, Yan SB, Williams MD, Graham DE, Nelson DR, Levy H, Bernard GR. Systemic host responses in severe sepsis analyzed by causative microorganism and treatment effects of drotrecogin alfa (activated). *Clin. Infect. Dis.* 2003; 37:50-58.

[40] Ince C, Sinaasappel M. Microcirculatory oxygenation and shunting in sepsis and shock. *Crit Care Med.* 1999; 27:1369-1377.

[41] Petros A, Bennett D, Vallance P. Effect of nitric oxide synthase inhibitors on hypotension in patients with septic shock. *Lancet.* 1991; 338:1557-1558.

[42] Marshall J. Inflammation, coagulopathy, and the pathogenesis of multiple organ dysfunction syndrome. *Crit. Care Med.* 2001; 29:S99-S106.

[43] Harlan JM. Leukocyte-endothelial interactions. *Blood.* 1985; 65:513-525.

[44] Deshpande SS, Angkeow P, Huang J, Ozaki M, Irani K. Rac1 inhibits TNF-alpha-induced endothelial cell apoptosis: dual regulation by reactive oxygen species. *FASEB J.* 2000; 14:1705-1714.

[45] Damle NK, Doyle LV, Bender JR, Bradley EC. Interleukin 2-activated human lymphocytes exhibit enhanced adhesion to normal vascular endothelial cells and cause their lysis. *J. Immunol.* 1987; 138:1779-1785.

[46] Haeney MR. The role of the complement cascade in sepsis. *J Antimicrob Chemother.* 1998; 41 (Suppl A):41-46.

[47] Walport MJ. Complement. First of two parts. *N. Engl. J. Med.* 2001; 344:1058-1066.
[48] Ward PA. Sepsis, apoptosis and complement. *Biochem. Pharmacol.* 2008; 76:1383-1388.
[49] Ho YP, Sheen IS, Chiu CT, Wu CS, Lin CY. A strong association between down-regulation of HLA-DR expression and the late mortality in patients with severe acute pancreatitis. *Am. J. Gastroenterol.* 2006; 101:1117-1124.
[50] Monneret G, Lepape A, Voirin N, Bohe J, Venet F, Debard AL, Thizy H, Bienvenu J, Gueyffier F, Vanhems P. Persisting low monocyte human leukocyte antigen-DR expression predicts mortality in septic shock. *Intensive Care Med.* 2006; 32:1175-1183.
[51] Pachot A, Lepape A, Vey S, Bienvenu J, Mougin B, Monneret G. Systemic transcriptional analysis in survivor and nonsurvivor septic shock patients: a preliminary study. *Immunol. Lett.* 2006; 106:63-71.
[52] Hall MW, Gavrilin MA, Knatz NL, Duncan MD, Fernandez SA, Wewers MD. Monocyte mRNA phenotype and adverse outcomes from pediatric multiple organ dysfunction syndrome. *Pediatr. Res.* 2007; 62:597-603.
[53] Bohuslav J, Kravchenko VV, Parry GC, Erlich JH, Gerondakis S, Mackman N, Ulevitch RJ. Regulation of an essential innate immune response by the p50 subunit of NF-kappaB. *J. Clin. Invest.* 1998; 102:1645-1652.
[54] Wahlstrom K, Bellingham J, Rodriguez JL, West MA. Inhibitory kappaB alpha control of nuclear factor-kappaB is dysregulated in endotoxin tolerant macrophages. *Shock.* 1999; 11:242-247.
[55] Medvedev AE, Lentschat A, Wahl LM, Golenbock DT, Vogel SN. Dysregulation of LPS-induced Toll-like receptor 4-MyD88 complex formation and IL-1 receptor-associated kinase 1 activation in endotoxin-tolerant cells. *J. Immunol.* 2002; 169:5209-5216.
[56] Fumeaux T, Pugin J. Role of interleukin-10 in the intracellular sequestration of human leukocyte antigen-DR in monocytes during septic shock. *Am. J. Respir. Crit. Care Med.* 2002; 166:1475-1482.
[57] Le Tulzo Y, Pangault C, Amiot L, Guilloux V, Tribut O, Arvieux C, Camus C, Fauchet R, Thomas R, Drénou B. Monocyte human leukocyte antigen-DR transcriptional downregulation by cortisol during septic shock. *Am. J. Respir. Crit. Care Med.* 2004; 169:1144-1151.

[58] Volk T, Schmutzler M, Engelhardt L, Döcke WD, Volk HD, Konertz W, Kox WJ. Influence of aminosteroid and glucocorticoid treatment on inflammation and immune function during cardiopulmonary bypass. *Crit. Care Med.* 2001; 29:2137-2142.

[59] Hotchkiss RS, Tinsley KW, Swanson PE, Chang KC, Cobb JP, Buchman TG, Korsmeyer SJ, Karl IE. Prevention of lymphocyte cell death in sepsis improves survival in mice. *Proc. Natl. Acad. Sci. U S A.* 1999; 96:14541-14546.

[60] Volk HD, Reinke P, Docke WD. Clinical aspects: from systemic inflammation to 'immunoparalysis'. *Chem. Immunol.* 2000; 74:162-177.

[61] Hall MW, Knatz NL, Vetterly C, Tomarello S, Wewers MD, Volk HD, Carcillo JA. Immunoparalysis and nosocomial infection in children with multiple organ dysfunction syndrome. *Intensive Care Med.* 2011; 37:525-532.

[62] Calvin JE, Driedger AA, Sibbald WJ. An assessment of myocardial function in human sepsis utilizing ECG gated cardiac scintigraphy. *Chest.* 1981; 80:579-586.

[63] Parker MM, Shelhamer JH, Bacharach SL, Green MV, Natanson C, Frederick TM, Damske BA, Parrillo JE. Profound but reversible myocardial depression in patients with septic shock. *Ann. Intern. Med.* 1984; 100:483-490.

[64] Charpentier J, Luyt CE, Fulla Y, Vinsonneau C, Cariou A, Grabar S, Dhainaut JF, Mira JP, Chiche JD. Brain natriuretic peptide: A marker of myocardial dysfunction and prognosis during severe sepsis. *Crit. Care Med.* 2004; 32:660-665.

[65] Cunnion RE, Schaer GL, Parker MM, Natanson C, Parrillo JE. The coronary circulation in human septic shock. *Circulation.* 1986; 73: 637-644.

[66] Herbertson MJ, Werner HA, Russell JA, Iversen K, Walley KR. Myocardial oxygen extraction ratio is decreased during endotoxemia in pigs. *J. Appl. Physiol.* 1995; 79:479-486.

[67] Dhainaut JF, Huyghebaert MF, Monsallier JF, Lefevre G, Dall'Ava-Santucci J, Brunet F, Villemant D, Carli A, Raichvarg D. Coronary hemodynamics and myocardial metabolism of lactate, free fatty acids, glucose, and ketones in patients with septic shock. *Circulation.* 1987; 75:533-541.

[68] Solomon MA, Correa R, Alexander HR, Koev LA, Cobb JP, Kim DK, Roberts WC, Quezado ZM, Scholz TD, Cunnion RE, Hoffman WD, Bacher J, Yatsiv I, Natanson C. Myocardial energy metabolism and morphology in a canine model of sepsis. *Am. J. Physiol.* 1994; 266:H757-H768.

[69] Van Lambalgen AA, van Kraats AA, Mulder MF, Teerlink T, van den Bos GC. High-energy phosphates in heart, liver, kidney, and skeletal muscle of endotoxemic rats. *Am J Physiol.* 1994; 266:H1581-H1587.

[70] Levy RJ, Piel DA, Acton PD, Zhou R, Ferrari VA, Karp JS, Deutschman CS. Evidence of myocardial hibernation in the septic heart. *Crit. Care Med.* 2005; 33:2752-2756.

[71] Parrillo JE, Burch C, Shelhamer JH, Parker MM, Natanson C, Schuette W. A circulating myocardial depressant substance in humans with septic shock: septic shock patients with a reduced ejection fraction have a circulating factor that depresses in vitro myocardial cell performance. *J. Clin. Invest.* 1985; 76:1539-1553.

[72] Mink SN, Jacobs H, Duke K, Bose D, Cheng ZQ, Light RB. N, N', N'' -triacetylglucosamine, an inhibitor of lysozyme, prevents myocardial depression in Escherichia coli sepsis in dogs. *Crit. Care Med.* 2004; 32:184-193.

[73] Konrad D, Oldner A, Rossi P, Wanecek M, Rudehill A, Weitzberg E. Differentiated and dose-related cardiovascular effects of a dual endothelin receptor antagonist in endotoxin shock. *Crit. Care Med.* 2004; 32:1192-1199.

[74] Massion PB, Feron O, Dessy C, Balligand JL. Nitric oxide and cardiac function: ten years after, and continuing. *Circ Res.* 2003; 93:388-398.

[75] Reines HD, Halushka PV, Cook JA, Wise WC, Rambo W. Plasma thromboxane concentrations are raised in patients dying with septic shock. *Lancet.* 1982; 2:174-175.

[76] Cines DB, Pollak ES, Buck CA, Loscalzo J, Zimmerman GA, McEver RP, Pober JS, Wick TM, Konkle BA, Schwartz BS, Barnathan ES, McCrae KR, Hug BA, Schmidt AM, Stern DM. Endothelial cells in physiology and in the pathophysiology of vascular disorders. *Blood.* 1998; 91:3527-3561.

[77] Gross SS, Kilbourn RG, Griffith OW. NO in septic shock: Good, bad or ugly? Learning from iNOS knockouts. *Trends Microbiol.* 1996; 4:47-49.

[78] Chagnon F, Bentourkia Mh, Lecomte R, Lessard M, Lesur O. Endotoxin-induced heart dysfunction in rats: Assessment of myocardial perfusion and permeability and the role of fluid resuscitation. *Crit. Care Med.* 2006; 34:127-133.

[79] Maitland K, Kiguli S, Opoka RO, Engoru C, Olupot-Olupot P, Akech SO, Nyeko R, Mtove G, Reyburn H, Lang T, Brent B, Evans JA, Tibenderana JK, Crawley J, Russell EC, Levin M, Babiker AG, Gibb DM; FEAST Trial Group. Mortality after Fluid Bolus in African Children with Severe Infection. *N. Engl. J. Med.* 2011; 364:2483-2495.

INDEX

A

Abraham, 115, 123, 124, 125
access, 5, 37, 62
access device, 62
accounting, 79
acetylcholine, 11
acid, 53, 61, 63, 67, 140, 144
acidic, 124
acidosis, 4, 20, 32, 56, 58, 112
ACTH, 38, 105, 107
acute lung injury, 30, 35, 46, 125, 144
acute organ dysfunction, x, 119
acute respiratory distress syndrome, 35, 57
adaptation, 18
adenine, 53, 146
adenosine, vii, 1, 4, 16, 20, 22, 25, 128
adenosine triphosphate, 128
adhesion, 11, 42, 53, 96, 112, 132, 133, 134, 136, 146
adipose, 63, 102
adipose tissue, 63, 102
adjustment, 11
ADP, 7, 16, 21
adults, viii, 9, 14, 23, 27, 32, 42, 46, 49, 54, 55, 56, 81, 82, 110, 138, 139
adverse effects, 86, 108
adverse event, ix, 38, 76, 80, 86, 88
aetiology, 90

age, ix, xi, 29, 41, 56, 57, 76, 87, 88, 127, 128, 142
agencies, 59
aggregation, 136
agonist, 18
agranulocytosis, vii, ix, 76, 77, 78, 79, 80, 81, 82, 83, 84, 85, 86, 87, 88, 89, 90, 91
albumin, 38
algorithm, 60
ALI, 35
alkalosis, 32
alters, 3
alveolar type II cells, 23
amines, 137
amino, 63, 124
amino acids, 124
aminoglycosides, 85
amplitude, 3
anemia, 106, 115
anesthetics, 56
anorexia, 125
antibiotic, viii, 36, 37, 39, 41, 47, 48, 51, 78, 85, 86, 87, 120
antibiotic resistance, 85
antibody, 85, 123, 137
anticoagulant, 136
antidiuretic hormone, 139
antigen, 34, 131, 132, 137, 138
anti-inflammatory agents, 79
antimicrobial therapy, 37, 48

Index

antioxidant, 8, 66, 67, 68, 69, 70, 73, 74
anuria, 35
aorta, 111
APC, 37
aplastic anemia, 90
apoptosis, 7, 15, 17, 23, 123, 131, 133, 137, 138, 141, 145, 146, 147
ARDS, 35, 46, 57
arrest, 82
arterial blood gas, 34
arteries, 4, 95
arterioles, ix, 20, 93, 95, 98, 99, 101, 102, 110, 141
arteriovenous shunt, 96
artery, 35, 43, 46, 103, 140
aspergillosis, 84
assessment, 12, 35, 43, 55, 58, 64, 89, 97, 110, 112, 113, 148
asymptomatic, 81
ATP, 4, 7, 16, 20, 68, 128
attachment, 19
authorities, 55
autonomic nervous system, 19
autopsy, 16
aversion, 125
avoidance, 90
awareness, vii, viii, 27, 59, 70, 78

B

bacteremia, 41, 44, 48, 60, 65
bacteria, 8, 9, 29, 30, 37, 72, 132, 133, 137
bacterial infection, 32, 61, 64, 82, 132
bacterium, 8
baroreceptor, 139
barriers, 6, 21
base, 2, 61, 71
beneficial effect, 122
bicarbonate, 32, 47
bilirubin, 36, 57, 60, 69
binding, 121
bioavailability, 136
biochemistry, 73
biological markers, 33
biological processes, 63
biomarkers, ix, 45, 52, 59, 62, 63, 65, 67, 68, 69, 72, 73
biomolecules, 68
bleeding, 37, 106
blood cultures, 34, 62
blood dyscrasias, 89
blood flow, 4, 10, 11, 15, 22, 31, 35, 95, 99, 101, 102, 104, 108, 111, 113, 114, 115, 133, 136, 140, 146
blood pressure, 5, 7, 18, 19, 35, 36, 44, 53, 56, 57, 58, 103, 114, 136, 139, 141, 142
blood smear, 45
blood transfusion, 115
blood vessels, ix, 93, 95, 135
bloodstream, viii, 12, 48, 51, 62, 65, 132
body fluid, 63
body mass index (BMI), 38, 39, 102
body weight, 38, 39
bone, 81, 82
bone marrow, 81, 82
bowel, 57
bowel sounds, 57
brain, 25, 125
breathing, 34

C

C reactive protein, 56, 62, 65
Ca^{2+}, 3, 123
calcitonin, 63
calcium, viii, 2, 3, 4, 5, 6, 15, 21, 104, 123, 141
cancer, 55, 61, 71, 80
cancer XE "cancer" therapy, 55
capillary, x, 10, 57, 94, 95, 106, 107, 129, 134, 136, 146
capillary refill, 57
carbon, 112
carbon dioxide, 112
carboxyl, 15
cardiac enzymes, 16
cardiac muscle, 3, 4
cardiac operations, 112

Index

cardiac output, 2, 7, 9, 10, 12, 31, 35, 43, 44, 103, 139
cardiogenic shock, x, 10, 119
cardiomyopathy, vii, 1, 2, 26
cardiopulmonary bypass, 138, 148
cardiovascular system, 19, 108, 122
carotene, 68, 69
cascades, 134
caspases, 15
catecholamines, 4, 16, 18, 20, 107, 139
catheter, 34, 35, 46, 62
causal relationship, 139
causality, 89
cell, xi, 120, 123
cell death, 2, 13, 15, 134, 135, 138, 140, 148
cell killing, 137
cell surface, 131
challenges, 59
channel blocker, 4
chemical, 95
chemokines, 131, 132, 133, 134
chemotaxis, 139
chemotherapy, 77, 80, 85, 86, 89, 90, 91, 132
chest radiography, 40
children, 14, 24, 25, 45, 56, 57, 58, 64, 123, 128, 129, 138, 139, 142, 143, 148
Chile, 51, 127
China, 59
chronic illness, 98, 99
circulation, vii, 1, 9, 31, 35, 148
City, 75, 119
classes, 4, 29, 78, 131
cleavage, 15
clinical application, 26
clinical assessment, 113
clinical interventions, 59
clinical judgment, 59
clinical presentation, 80
clinical symptoms, viii, 27
clinical trials, xi, 31, 47, 122, 127, 129
closure, 4
clozapine, 78, 83

clustering, 135
CO_2, 97
coagulopathy, 134, 146
coma, 36, 52, 57
combined effect, 139
communication, xi, 95, 127, 129
community, 41, 46
complement, 12, 130, 133, 134, 137, 138, 146, 147
compliance, 39
complications, 35, 49, 72, 76, 83, 87, 112, 135
composition, 138
compounds, 141
comprehension, 142
conductance, 5
conference, 42, 47, 54, 56, 70, 129, 143
conjunctiva, 100
connectivity, 145
consensus, xi, 28, 38, 56, 59, 70, 77, 89, 127, 129, 143
Consensus, 41, 54, 56, 70, 143
constituents, 131
consumption, 31, 97, 106, 135
contamination, 100
control, xi, 120
control group, 86
controlled trials, 28
controversial, 66, 104
COPD, 38
coronary artery disease, 13
correlation, 7, 14, 17, 32, 43, 67
correlation coefficient, 32
corticosteroids, 20, 38, 107
cortisol, 138, 147
cost, 55, 87, 94
counterbalance, 138
covering, 102
creatine, 17
creatinine, 32, 36, 57, 58, 62, 82
CRIT, 115
CRP, 52, 56, 62, 64, 65, 69, 75
crystal structure, 7
CSF, ix, 76, 86, 87, 88, 91
culture, 34, 62, 64, 85

cuticle, 99
cycles, 66
cycling, 6
cyclooxygenase, 19, 136
cysteine, 4
cytochrome, 7, 25, 102
cytokines, 3, 6, 8, 9, 12, 13, 65, 66, 121, 130, 131, 132, 133, 134, 135, 136, 137, 140, 141, 142, 145
cytoplasm, 5, 131
cytoskeleton, 5, 6, 20

D

danger, 131, 144
death, 120
deaths, 128, 129, 142
debridement, 63
defects, 11
defense mechanisms, 130
deficiencies, 38, 45
deficiency, 45, 83
deficit, ix, x, 61, 71, 93, 94, 96, 109
deformability, 96, 111
degradation, 15, 52
dendritic cell, 131
depolarization, 95, 123
deposition, 96
deposits, 135
depression, vii, 1, 3, 7, 8, 11, 12, 13, 15, 16, 17, 22, 24, 31, 35, 139, 140, 141, 142, 148, 149
deprivation, 42, 43
derivatives, 67, 97
desensitization, 19
detectable, 8
detection, 41, 132, 144
developing countries, 128
diabetes, 29, 38, 39, 56, 99
diabetic patients, 35, 37
diagnostic criteria, 54
diastolic blood pressure, 19
differential diagnosis, 81
dilation, vii, 1
direct cost, 55

direct costs, 55
direct observation, 10
disease progression, 71
diseases, 29, 58, 63, 130, 142
disorder, ix, 18, 28, 76, 78, 81, 88
disseminated intravascular coagulation, 33, 45, 61, 130, 135
distress, ix, x, 10, 11, 58, 93, 94, 97, 109, 117
distribution, 10, 25, 31, 108
distributive shock, 2, 22, 31
DNA, xi, 16, 18, 120, 121, 124, 125
DNase, 124
dogs, 149
donors, 68
doppler, 99
dosage, 19
down-regulation, 147
drainage, 63
drug reactions, 89
drugs, ix, 76, 77, 78, 79, 81, 83, 90, 95
dyes, 98

E

E.coli, 7
edema, 11, 20, 56, 102, 113, 136
electron, 7, 17
emergency, 44, 45, 47, 60, 64, 71
EMS, 52, 60
encephalopathy, 34
endocrine, 130
endothelial cells, viii, ix, 7, 20, 31, 51, 66, 93, 95, 111, 130, 135, 136, 146
endothelial dysfunction, 11
endothelium, 31, 42, 95, 110, 111, 133, 134, 135, 136, 137, 141, 145
endotoxemia, 6, 17, 25, 112, 116, 121, 148
end-stage renal disease, 13
energy, 4, 15, 16, 17, 23, 49, 140, 149
England, 89
enrollment, xi, 58, 127, 129
environment, 66, 95
enzyme, 16, 19, 67, 73, 137, 141

Index

enzymes, 15, 68, 133, 134
epidemiologic, 29
epidemiology, 41, 70, 71, 89, 94, 110, 123, 143
epinephrine, 57
epithelia, 5
epithelial cells, 5, 20, 23
epithelium, x, 94
equipment, 98
erythrocytes, ix, 93
ESR, 58, 61
ESRD, 13, 23
etiology, 2, 37, 59, 61
eukaryotic, 16, 121, 131
eukaryotic cell, 16, 121, 131
Europe, 54, 78
evidence, viii, xi, 2, 3, 4, 7, 11, 12, 15, 17, 18, 19, 20, 28, 29, 34, 35, 37, 40, 48, 49, 64, 67, 85, 86, 88, 120, 129, 133, 135, 140, 141, 142
evolution, 66, 80, 139
excitation, 3
exotoxins, 9
exposure, 6, 16, 77
extraction, ix, x, 32, 93, 94, 96, 109, 140, 148

F

failure, x, 119, 123
families, 79, 131, 133
fatty acids, 148
fear, 37
fever, 32, 72, 80, 81, 83, 84, 85, 129, 134
fibrin, 61, 96, 135
fibrin degradation products, 61
fibrinogen, 61
fibrinolysis, 95
fibrinolytic, 130, 136
fluid, viii, 5, 6, 12, 21, 30, 33, 34, 35, 38, 46, 51, 56, 57, 58, 61, 69, 105, 106, 107, 128, 129, 139, 142, 150
fluid balance, 56
fluorescence, 112

football, 95
force, 6, 133
formation, 15, 19, 96, 135, 147
France, 75, 89
free radicals, xi, 16, 128
functional changes, 135
funding, 88
fungi, 8, 85

G

gangrene, 85
gastric mucosa, 36
gastrointestinal tract, 84
gene, xi, 120
gene expression, xi, 64, 120
genes, 16, 18, 65, 132, 135, 136, 138
genetic defect, 29, 41
genetics, 59, 130
genome, 64
gingival, 98
glucocorticoid, 148
glucose, 37, 47, 56, 58, 61, 120, 140, 148
glutamine, 69
glutathione, 68, 74
glycolysis, 16
gram negative organisms, 62
granules, 33
growth, ix, 76, 82, 86, 87, 88, 91
growth factor, ix, 76, 82, 86, 87, 88, 91
guidelines, 34, 36, 38, 42, 46, 48, 54, 63, 70, 71, 72, 108, 114, 142, 143

H

half-life, 64, 65, 67
health, 52, 54, 58, 59, 60, 61, 99, 102
health care, 54, 59
heart failure, 123
heart rate, 8, 9, 15, 19, 23, 25, 44, 60, 103
heart valves, 29
hematocrit, 33, 61

heme, 67
hemoglobin, 31, 33, 98, 100, 102, 106, 113
hemorrhage, 44
hemostasis, 95, 145
hepatocytes, 65
heterogeneity, x, 7, 10, 11, 94, 98, 101
High-mobility group protein B1 (HMGB1), xi, 120, 121
histone, 121
history, 37, 38, 39, 40, 71, 77, 81, 83
HIV, 5, 29, 52, 55
HIV-1, 5
HLA, 131, 138, 139, 147
homeostasis, 58
hormones, 21
hospitalization, 14, 87
host, viii, xi, 8, 24, 31, 38, 51, 59, 62, 120, 127, 129, 130, 131, 132, 134, 137, 146
human, 5, 17, 19, 22, 23, 25, 26, 37, 44, 48, 63, 64, 95, 101, 105, 108, 112, 113, 114, 116, 120, 123, 124, 138, 145, 146, 147, 148
human body, 95
human leukocyte antigen, 147
human neutrophils, 145
human skin, 113
human subjects, 108
Hunter, 2, 8, 12, 23, 71, 144
hydrocortisone, 38, 48, 107, 116
hydrogen, 16, 68, 133
hydrogen peroxide, 16, 68, 133
hydroxyl, 16, 68
hygiene, 84
hyperglycemia, 61, 125
hypersensitivity, 59
hypersplenism, 82
hypertension, 35
hyperthermia, 58
hyperventilation, 32
hypoglycemia, 37, 40
hypotension, 2, 3, 4, 10, 30, 32, 35, 48, 56, 57, 58, 80, 103, 129, 139, 146
hypotensive, 18, 114
hypothermia, 44
hypovolemia, 5, 6, 20, 33
hypoxemia, 57
hypoxia, ix, 4, 10, 15, 28, 31, 32, 36, 44, 93, 116, 130, 135, 136

I

ICAM, 53, 62
ICC, 70
ID, 145
ideal, 110
identification, viii, 28, 33, 36, 52, 58, 60, 62, 101
idiopathic, vii, ix, 76
idiosyncratic, ix, 76, 77, 78, 80, 82, 83, 85, 86, 87, 88, 89, 90, 91
IFN, 134
IL-13, 19, 20
IL-6, 121, 125
IL-8, 9, 12, 62, 64, 67, 69
illumination, 100
image, 80, 100, 101
immune function, 138, 139, 144, 148
immune response, 130, 131, 134, 137, 138, 144, 147
immune system, 9, 29, 120, 130, 131, 132, 133, 137
immunity, 95, 130
immunodeficiency, 52
immunoglobulin, 33, 122, 125
immunoglobulin superfamily, 33
immunosuppression, 55, 130, 138
immunotherapy, 77
impairments, 7
improvements, 55
in vitro, 5, 12, 13, 17, 25, 37, 43, 123, 149
in vivo, 20, 97, 113, 137
incidence, 36, 41, 54, 55, 78, 89, 90, 94, 110
independent variable, 86
India, 143
individualization, 103
individuals, 32, 81

inducer, 18
induction, 42, 134, 137
infant mortality, 128
infants, 25
inflammation, xi, 22, 24, 31, 61, 65, 66, 67, 72, 73, 120, 122, 125, 127, 129, 130, 132, 133, 134, 135, 137, 141, 145, 148
inflammatory disease, 65
inflammatory mediators, vii, viii, 1, 3, 8, 12, 21, 31, 51, 120, 135
inflammatory responses, 132
infrared spectroscopy, 98, 101, 102, 105, 113, 114, 115
inhibition, 5, 6, 7, 15, 17, 19, 21, 23, 138
inhibitor, viii, 2, 4, 5, 7, 22, 43, 85, 136, 138, 149
initiation, 8, 28, 37, 48, 60, 131
innate immunity, 144
institutions, 60
insulin, 37, 47, 125
integrin, 135, 136
integrins, 133
integrity, 13, 31, 99
intensive care unit, xi, 2, 42, 47, 48, 53, 64, 71, 108, 110, 120, 127, 128, 129
interactions, x, 119
intercellular adhesion molecule, 11, 136
interference, 5, 19
interferon, 9, 12, 77, 134
interferon gamma, 9, 12
internalization, 138
intervention, 34, 36, 58, 63, 80, 98, 101
intracellular calcium, 4
intravenous fluids, 35
ion channels, vii, 1, 3, 20, 21
iron, 17
irritability, 139
ischemia, x, 10, 15, 31, 94, 102, 103, 114, 140
isolation, 84

J

Japan, 27, 119

K

ketones, 148
kidney, 62, 149
killer cells, 53
kinetics, 11

L

laboratory tests, 58, 59
lactate level, 32, 33, 36, 44, 45, 97, 103, 112
lactic acid, 4, 30, 32, 33, 35, 43, 47, 106
landscape, 10
L-arginine, viii, 2, 7, 17
lead, viii, ix, 11, 27, 28, 58, 59, 69, 93, 96, 120, 132, 136
leakage, 5, 6, 13, 15, 61
LED, 113
left ventricle, 125
lens, 100
leukocytes, viii, 51, 136
leukocytosis, 61
leukopenia, 33, 61
ligand, 136
light, 5, 16, 20, 38, 53, 62, 99, 100, 101
light emitting diode, 100
lipid peroxidation, 68, 73
lipids, 68
lipoproteins, 111
liver, 29, 30, 32, 36, 38, 39, 58, 61, 63, 97, 149
liver disease, 29, 38, 39
liver enzymes, 32, 36, 58, 61
localization, xi, 61, 120
low risk, 72, 83
low temperatures, 32
lycopene, 69
lymphocytes, 132, 146
lymphoid, 138
lysine, xi, 120
lysis, 8, 133, 137, 146
lysozyme, 140, 149

M

machinery, 3
macrophages, 8, 12, 31, 121, 131, 137, 145, 147
magnitude, 4, 59
major histocompatibility complex, 128, 131, 132
majority, 76, 78, 81
malaise, 80
malignancy, 29
malnutrition, 38, 39, 49
man, 43
management, vii, viii, ix, 27, 28, 33, 34, 35, 37, 39, 40, 42, 46, 49, 62, 71, 72, 73, 76, 78, 81, 82, 83, 85, 88, 89, 90, 91, 94, 97, 106, 107, 108, 114
marrow, 81
mass, 38, 39
matrix, 7, 17
matter, iv, 15, 22, 24, 109
mean arterial pressure, 36
measurement, 12, 13, 14, 33, 43, 44, 95, 97, 98, 101, 111, 112, 139
mechanical ventilation, 34, 38, 42, 56, 57, 60
medical, ix, 29, 49, 52, 55, 60, 71, 78, 80, 81, 83, 93, 111, 116
medical history, 29, 81
Medicare, 41
medication, 79, 81, 83
medicine, 44, 72, 73, 85, 86, 88, 143, 144
memory, 137
meningococcemia, 29, 45
messages, 133
meta-analysis, 64
Metabolic, 21
metabolic acidosis, 3, 33, 57, 61
metabolic disorders, ix, 76, 88, 142
metabolism, 11, 15, 16, 36, 68, 97, 141, 148, 149
metabolites, 77
methylene blue, 17
methylprednisolone, 138

MHC, 128
mice, 6, 17, 43, 124, 148
microcirculation, vii, ix, x, 1, 10, 11, 21, 24, 93, 94, 95, 96, 97, 99, 100, 101, 102, 103, 104, 105, 106, 107, 108, 109, 111, 112, 113, 115, 116, 136, 141
microorganisms, 29, 39, 131, 146
microscope, 99
microscopy, 6, 13, 97, 101, 112, 113
migration, 134
misuse, 79
mitochondria, 3, 6, 8, 21, 68, 109, 146
mitochondrial DNA, 18
mitogen, 121
mobility, xi, 120, 121, 122, 124, 125
model, 125
models, 10, 12, 15, 17, 20, 60, 66, 140, 142
modifications, 67
molecules, 11, 42, 68, 78, 96, 131, 132, 133, 134, 136, 138, 141
monoclonal antibody, 123
morbidity, x, xi, 18, 21, 31, 33, 38, 40, 69, 119, 127, 128, 129, 138
morphology, 149
mortality rate, vii, viii, ix, 27, 28, 37, 39, 55, 76, 82, 86, 87, 88, 95, 120, 128, 140
motif, 124
movement, 123
mRNA, 147
mucormycosis, 84
mucosa, 98, 100
multivariate analysis, 82, 86
muscle mass, 38
myelodysplasia, 86
myelodysplastic syndromes, 82
myeloid cells, 33, 46, 81, 82
myelosuppression, 91
myocardial infarction, 15, 43
myocardial necrosis, 15, 140
myocardium, 3, 6, 12, 13, 15, 16, 17, 140, 141
myocyte, 6, 8, 12, 15, 17, 121, 140

myoglobin, 102
myosin, 5, 6, 16

N

Na$^+$, 5, 23
NAD, 16
National Institutes of Health, 53
natural killer cell, 73, 131, 137
necrosis, 7, 20, 53, 121, 123
neonates, 111
Netherlands, 90
neurons, 3, 4
neutropenia, ix, 33, 61, 76, 77, 78, 80, 81, 82, 83, 84, 85, 86, 88, 90, 91, 132
neutrophils, 8, 31, 45, 64, 67, 68, 96, 97, 111, 130, 132, 133, 136, 137, 139
NHS, 1
nicotinamide, 146
nitric oxide, vii, 1, 3, 4, 7, 9, 11, 16, 20, 21, 23, 68, 107, 123, 128, 133, 134, 136, 141, 146
nitric oxide synthase, 3, 4, 9, 11, 21, 128, 134, 136, 146
nitrite, 17, 24, 67
nitrogen, viii, 16, 51, 52, 53, 58, 62, 66, 68, 128, 133
NK cells, 53, 66, 70
norepinephrine, 57, 103, 114
North America, 30
NRS, 38
nucleosome, xi, 120, 121
nucleotides, 123
nucleus, xi, 120, 121, 132
nutrients, 95, 108, 135
nutrition, 38, 39, 40, 48, 49
nutritional deficiencies, 82
nutritional status, 38, 130

O

obstruction, 97
occlusion, 99, 103
oil, 99

optimization, 28
organelles, 6
organism, x, 18, 22, 33, 62, 119, 132
organs, 30, 31, 35, 100, 120, 121, 138
outpatient, 63
oxidation, 4, 67
oxidation products, 67
oxidative damage, 67, 68, 70
oxidative stress, xi, 66, 67, 70, 128, 132, 141, 142, 144
oxygen, ix, 2, 7, 10, 11, 15, 16, 23, 31, 32, 34, 36, 42, 43, 44, 46, 47, 53, 56, 66, 68, 93, 94, 95, 96, 97, 102, 103, 104, 105, 106, 109, 112, 113, 128, 134, 135, 136, 137, 140, 142, 148
oxygen consumption, 11, 23, 31, 102, 103, 105, 106
oxyhemoglobin, 35, 36, 99

P

pancreatitis, 147
paralysis, 2, 130, 139
patents, 40
pathogenesis, vii, xi, 1, 2, 8, 10, 17, 25, 38, 110, 121, 127, 129, 130, 132, 145, 146
pathogens, 29, 130, 131, 133, 134
pathology, ix, 52, 69, 81, 136
pathophysiological, vii, ix, 1, 3, 52, 70, 142
pathophysiology, vii, xi, 10, 30, 55, 67, 70, 71, 91, 107, 127, 129, 135, 140, 142, 145, 149
pathways, 6, 16, 17, 21, 121, 123, 130, 132, 136, 137, 140, 145
patient care, xi, 127, 129
pattern recognition, 131
PCT, 53, 56, 62, 63, 64, 65, 69
peptide, 5, 13, 63, 133, 148
peptides, 5, 72, 131
performance, 123
perfusion, vii, x, 1, 9, 11, 21, 26, 34, 35, 36, 58, 94, 96, 97, 98, 99, 101, 103,

104, 106, 107, 108, 113, 114, 116, 136, 139, 142, 146, 150
perineum, 84
peripheral blood, 61
peritonitis, 60
permeability, 5, 9, 20, 42, 66, 136, 137, 141, 150
permit, xi, 127
peroxidation, 67, 68
peroxide, 128
peroxynitrite, 5, 7, 16, 17, 21, 26, 68, 128, 141
personal history, 58
petechiae, 58
phagocytic cells, 137
phagocytosis, 130, 131, 137, 139, 145
phenotype, 147
phenotypes, 111
phenylalanine, 133
phosphate, 15, 53, 140, 146
phosphates, 149
phosphorylation, vii, 1, 5, 6, 7, 20, 21, 24, 123
phototoxicity, 112
physicians, 143
physiology, 31, 52, 145, 149
pigs, 111, 148
pilot study, 125
placebo, 4, 104, 105, 115, 123, 124
plasma levels, 9, 64
plasma membrane, 4, 131
plasma proteins, 137
plasminogen, 43, 136
platelet activating factor, 9
platelet aggregation, 142
platelet count, 36, 57
platelets, 60, 136
playing, ix, 93, 130, 135
pneumonia, ix, 41, 46, 60, 76, 80, 88
polarization, x, 10, 94, 99
policy, 37
polymerase, vii, 1, 16, 20, 25, 34
polymerase chain reaction, 34
polypeptides, 133
polysaccharide, 65

pools, 16
population, 13, 54, 64, 78, 89, 106, 107
positive correlation, 15, 16
positron, 11
positron emission tomography, 11
potassium, 4, 5, 20, 21
preparation, iv, 85, 88
prevention, viii, 5, 27, 84, 112, 133
priming, 133
principles, 34
probability, 60, 65
probe, 100, 102
production, 125
professionals, 59
prognosis, vii, ix, 1, 25, 33, 45, 63, 76, 83, 88, 97, 148
pro-inflammatory, 12, 64, 121, 133, 134, 135, 141
proliferation, 37, 67, 132
propagation, 3, 8
prophylactic, 84
prosthetic device, 29
prosthetic materials, 62
protection, 34
protein kinase C, 121
protein kinases, vii, 1, 5, 16, 121, 123
proteins, vii, 1, 3, 5, 6, 12, 13, 15, 16, 17, 19, 21, 61, 121, 124, 132
proteolytic enzyme, 133, 134
public health, xi, 127, 128
pulmonary edema, 20, 142
pulmonary vascular resistance, 9
purpura, 22, 26, 45

Q

quantification, 26, 98, 102

R

radicals, 134, 136
radiotherapy, 77
reactant, 53, 65, 67
reactants, 62

Index 161

reactions, 31
reactive oxygen, viii, 16, 51, 66, 68, 128, 133, 137, 145, 146
reactivity, 10, 78, 85, 98, 99, 103, 106, 114
reason, 121
receptors, vii, 1, 3, 6, 8, 19, 20, 21, 24, 31, 32, 41, 131, 137
recognition, 29, 31, 36, 39, 40, 41, 59, 60, 69, 82, 124, 129, 130, 131, 132, 144
recommendations, iv, 28, 38, 39, 40, 85
recovery, 12, 18, 69, 77, 82, 86, 87, 91, 140
recruiting, 134
rectal temperature, 32
red blood cells, 95, 96, 99, 106, 136
reflexes, 130, 139
regression, 65
regression analysis, 65
regulation, 121
relaxation, 4, 5, 6, 12, 24, 121
relevance, 2
reliability, 101
renaissance, 38
renal failure, ix, 76, 82, 88, 129
renin, 18, 139
repair, 120, 129
replication, 18
requirements, 5, 14, 57
residues, 4
resistance, 8, 9, 28, 37, 120, 134
resolution, 133
resources, 55
respiration, 7, 16, 32, 34, 44, 130, 141
respiratory rate, 29, 30
responsiveness, 4, 6, 16, 19, 23, 35, 46, 107, 139
restoration, 35, 36, 107
reticulum, 3
retinol, 69
rheumatoid arthritis, 64
ribose, vii, 1, 7, 16, 20, 21, 22, 25
risk, vii, viii, ix, 19, 27, 28, 29, 37, 38, 39, 40, 42, 52, 55, 60, 61, 63, 66, 69, 76, 77, 78, 79, 81, 83, 84, 85, 89, 110, 130, 133
risk factors, vii, viii, ix, 27, 28, 29, 42, 52, 60, 69, 89, 110
rituximab, 77
RNA, 53, 64
rodents, 138
ROOH, 68

S

safety, 41, 86
saliva, 101
Salmonella, 24, 82
saturation, 7, 31, 32, 35, 36, 43, 44, 46, 47, 53, 56, 97, 98, 102, 106, 113
scattering, 100
scientific knowledge, 2
scope, 108, 141
secretion, 62, 131, 137
sedatives, 108
sensing, 95
sensitivity, 6, 13, 14, 25, 32, 45, 61, 64, 65, 69, 129
Sepsis, x, 119, 120, 121, 123, 124
serum, 12, 13, 14, 21, 23, 32, 33, 36, 58, 60, 61, 62, 63, 65, 72, 82, 120, 121, 122, 123, 138, 140
services, iv, 52, 60, 71
shear, 133
showing, 6, 14, 64, 66, 82
signaling pathway, 121, 123, 132
signalling, 19, 42
signals, 131
signs, 32, 33, 35, 36, 58, 61, 80, 84, 134, 139
silver, 28, 41
skeletal muscle, 3, 4, 7, 111, 149
skin, 20, 34, 35, 58, 62, 80, 84, 98, 99, 100, 102, 112, 139
smooth muscle, vii, ix, 1, 4, 18, 19, 23, 25, 93, 95, 137
smooth muscle cells, ix, 4, 19, 23, 93, 95
society, 143
sodium, 5, 23, 60, 122, 125

solution, 107
species, viii, 16, 51, 53, 66, 68, 128, 133, 137, 145, 146
spectrophotometry, 7
spleen, 63
sputum, 80
stability, xi, 120, 121
stabilization, 11, 34
staphylococci, 9
starch, 107, 116
state, vii, 1, 6, 7, 10, 31, 32, 95, 100, 134, 135, 136, 138
states, 4, 5, 10, 135
sterile, 48, 62
steroids, 29, 38, 107, 120, 138
stimulation, 9, 19, 38, 134, 136, 137, 139
stimulus, 65
stomach, 112
stool culture, 84
stool cultures, 84
strategies, 120
stratification, 64
streptococci, 9
stress, x, 24, 67, 70, 73, 94, 129, 142
stress test, x, 94
stroke, 2, 8, 9, 14
stroke volume, 9
structural protein, 16
structure, xi, 7, 95, 120, 121, 131
substrate, 7
sulfonylurea, 4
Sun, 144
supervision, 84
suppression, xi, 127, 130, 138
surrogates, 38
survival, viii, 10, 36, 38, 44, 45, 47, 48, 52, 64, 65, 66, 69, 72, 108, 113, 132, 141, 148
survival rate, viii, 52, 69
survivors, 15, 16, 24, 25, 64, 65, 69, 74, 138, 140
susceptibility, 29, 38, 59, 130, 132
swelling, 7, 136
symptoms, vii, viii, 27, 58, 83, 134

syndrome, viii, 2, 27, 29, 30, 32, 40, 42, 51, 52, 53, 54, 55, 56, 58, 59, 71, 72, 73, 82, 109, 111, 117, 124, 128, 129, 130, 138, 143, 146, 147, 148
synthesis, 61, 62, 134
systemic lupus erythematosus, 82
systolic blood pressure, 60

T

T lymphocytes, 137
tachycardia, 32, 35, 129
tachypnea, 32, 129
target, ix, 35, 36, 52, 55, 60, 67, 73, 87, 95, 107, 108, 110, 122, 144
target population, 87
targets, 121
taste aversion, 125
techniques, ix, x, 10, 12, 28, 93, 94, 98, 100, 101, 103, 112
technologies, 97, 109
teicoplanin, 85
temperature, 29, 30, 32, 56, 57, 60, 98, 99
tension, 36, 112
tensions, 112
testing, 13, 34, 63
TGF, 19, 20
Thailand, 90
therapeutic agents, 38
therapeutic approaches, vii, 1, 2
therapeutic targets, 121
therapy, viii, 10, 11, 27, 28, 33, 36, 37, 38, 39, 40, 41, 46, 47, 48, 58, 60, 62, 63, 65, 85, 86, 87, 97, 104, 106, 110, 116, 120, 122, 125
thrombin, 122, 135, 136
thrombocytopenia, 30, 61, 89
thrombomodulin, 122
thrombosis, 31, 43, 145
thyroid, 63
tissue perfusion, ix, x, 94, 96, 106, 107, 108, 111
TLR, 131
TLR2, 122, 132

Index

TLR4, 122, 132, 138
TNF, 3, 5, 8, 9, 12, 13, 15, 16, 19, 21, 53, 62, 65, 67, 77, 121, 125, 128, 134, 136, 137, 139, 140, 142, 146
TNF-alpha, 146
TNF-α, 53, 62, 65, 67, 121, 134, 136, 137, 139, 140, 142
tonometry, 36, 97
tonsillitis, 80
toxic effect, 98
toxin, 9, 20
tracks, 22
trafficking, 10, 135
transcription, 16, 18, 19, 23, 62, 121, 123, 132, 135, 136, 138, 144, 146
transcription factors, 23, 62, 121, 123, 136, 144
transduction, 5, 132
transfusion, 33, 105, 106, 115
transmission, 3
transport, x, 7, 10, 17, 23, 31, 63, 94, 95, 96, 113
trauma, 34, 41, 64, 72, 129
trial, 22, 35, 37, 38, 46, 47, 48, 64, 107, 109, 110, 115, 123, 124
tuberculosis, 82
tumor, vii, 1, 20, 121, 123, 128, 134, 145
tumor necrosis factor, vii, 1, 121, 123, 128, 134, 145

U

UK, 1, 129
ultrasound, 14, 63
underlying mechanisms, 138
United, 41, 54, 94, 106, 110, 115, 120, 123, 128, 129, 143
United States (USA), 41, 54, 58, 62, 94, 106, 110, 115, 120, 123, 129, 143
unstable angina, 15
urea, 52
uric acid, 69
urinalysis, 40
urinary tract, 58, 62
urine, 36, 40, 57, 62, 84, 85

V

validation, 113
vancomycin, 85
variables, ix, 7, 24, 25, 47, 60, 82, 93, 97, 98, 101, 103, 104, 105, 106, 108, 109, 112
vascular occlusion, x, 94
vasculature, 3
vasoconstriction, 98, 99, 136
vasodilation, 4, 9, 141, 142
vasodilator, 11
vasomotor, 2, 10, 95, 135
vasopressor, 18, 19, 38, 99, 103
velocity, 10, 14, 140
ventilation, 53, 60
ventricle, 12, 125
venules, ix, 93, 95, 98, 99, 101, 102
vessels, 18, 98, 99, 100, 102
video microscopy, 10
viral infection, 64, 77, 82
vitamins, 68, 69, 73

W

Wales, 89
war, 60, 64
water, 68
weight loss, 38
white blood cell count, 90
WHO, 143
withdrawal, 83
worldwide, xi, 127, 128

Y

yield, 14, 37